ABC of
Kidney Disease

Second Edition

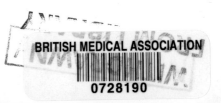

ABC series

An outstanding collection of resources – written by specialists for non-specialists

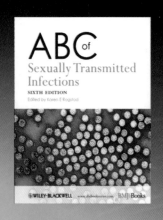

ABC of Sexually Transmitted Infections
SIXTH EDITION
Edited by Karen E Rogstad

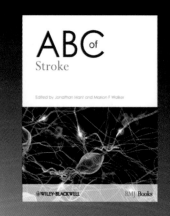

ABC of Stroke
Edited by Jonathan Mant and Marion F Walker

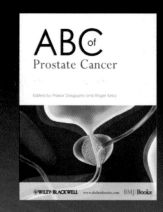

ABC of Prostate Cancer
Edited by Prokar Dasgupta and Roger Kirby

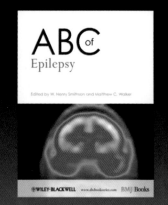

ABC of Epilepsy
Edited by W. Henry Smithson and Matthew C. Walker

The *ABC* series contains a wealth of indispensable resources for GPs, GP registrars, junior doctors, doctors in training and all those in primary care

- ▶ **Now fully revised and updated**
- ▶ **Highly illustrated, informative and a practical source of knowledge**
- ▶ **An easy-to-use resource, covering the symptoms, investigations, treatment and management of conditions presenting in day-to-day practice and patient support**
- ▶ **Full colour photographs and illustrations aid diagnosis and patient understanding of a condition**

For more information on all books in the *ABC* series, including links to further information, references and links to the latest official guidelines, please visit:

www.abcbookseries.com

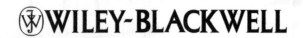

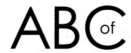

ABC of

Kidney Disease

Second Edition

David Goldsmith

Reader in Renal Medicine
School of Medicine and Dentistry
King's College London, London, UK

Satish Jayawardene

Consultant Nephrologist
King's College Hospital NHS Foundation Trust, London, UK

Penny Ackland

General Practitioner
Nunhead Surgery, Nunhead Grove, South East London, UK

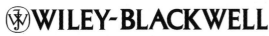

WILEY-BLACKWELL

A John Wiley & Sons, Ltd., Publication

BMJ|Books

This edition first published 2013 © 2013 John Wiley & Sons, Ltd

BMJ Books is an imprint of BMJ Publishing Group Limited, used under licence by Blackwell Publishing which was acquired by John Wiley & Sons in February 2007. Blackwell's publishing programme has been merged with Wiley's global Scientific, Technical and Medical business to form Wiley-Blackwell.

Registered office: John Wiley & Sons, Ltd, The Atrium, Southern Gate, Chichester, West Sussex, PO19 8SQ, UK

Editorial offices: 9600 Garsington Road, Oxford, OX4 2DQ, UK

The Atrium, Southern Gate, Chichester, West Sussex, PO19 8SQ, UK

111 River Street, Hoboken, NJ 07030-5774, USA

For details of our global editorial offices, for customer services and for information about how to apply for permission to reuse the copyright material in this book please see our website at www.wiley.com/wiley-blackwell.

Library of Congress Cataloging-in-Publication Data
ABC of kidney disease / [edited by] David Goldsmith, Satish Jayawardene, Penny Ackland. – 2nd ed.
p. ; cm. – (ABC series)
Includes bibliographical references and index.
ISBN 978-0-470-67204-4 (pbk. : alk. paper)
I. Goldsmith, David, 1959- II. Jayawardene, Satish. III. Ackland, Penny. IV.
Series: ABC series (Malden, Mass.)
[DNLM: 1. Kidney Diseases. 2. Kidney Failure, Chronic. WJ 300]

A catalogue record for this book is available from the British Library.

Wiley also publishes its books in a variety of electronic formats. Some content that appears in print may not be available in electronic books.

Cover image: PASIEKA/SCIENCE PHOTO LIBRARY
Cover design by Meaden Creative

Set in 9.25/12 Minion by Laserwords Private Limited, Chennai, India
Printed and bound in Malaysia by Vivar Printing Sdn Bhd

1   2013

Contents

Contributors

Penny Ackland
General Practitioner, Nunhead Surgery, Nunhead Grove, South East London, UK

Behdad Afzali
Wellcome Trust Senior Fellow in Nephrology, King's College London, London, UK

James O. Burton
NIHR Clinical Lecturer, Department of Infection, Immunity and Inflammation, School of Medicine and Biological Sciences, University of Leicester, Leicester, UK

Frances Coldstream
NIHR GSTFT/KCL Biomedical Research Centre, Guy's and St Thomas' NHS Foundation Trust, London, UK

John Feehally
Professor of Nephrology, The John Walls Renal Unit, Leicester General Hospital, Leicester, UK

Sean Gallagher
Senior House Officer, Renal Medicine, Guy's and St Thomas' NHS Foundation Trust, London, UK

David Goldsmith
Reader in Renal Medicine, School of Medicine and Dentistry, King's College London, London, UK

Irene Hadjimichael
Renal ST5, South Thames Rotation at King's College Hospital NHS Foundation Trust, London, UK

Ming He
Clinical Fellow in Transplant Surgery, Guy's and St Thomas' NHS Foundation Trust, London, UK

Rachel Hilton
Consultant Nephrologist, Guy's and St Thomas' NHS Foundation Trust, London, UK

Richard Hull
Specialist Registrar Nephrology, Guy's and St Thomas' NHS Foundation Trust, London, UK

Satish Jayawardene
Consultant Nephrologist, King's College Hospital NHS Foundation Trust, London, UK

Philip Kalra
Consultant Nephrologist and Honorary Professor of Nephrology, Hope Hospital, Salford, UK

Douglas Maclean
Former Renal Pharmacist, Guy's and St Thomas' NHS Foundation Trust, London, UK (deceased)

Christopher W. McIntyre
Reader in Vascular Medicine, Department of Renal Medicine, Derby City Hospital, Derby, UK

Emma Murphy
BRC PhD Clinical Research Training Fellow, NIHR GSTFT/KCL Biomedical Research Centre, Guy's and St Thomas' NHS Foundation Trust, London, UK Department of Palliative Care, Policy and Rehabilitation, Cicely Saunders Institute, King's College London, London, UK

Donal O' Donoghue
Consultant Renal Physician, Hope Hospital, Salford, UK National Clinical Director for Renal Services

Christopher Reid
Consultant Paediatric Nephrologist, Evelina Children's Hospital, Guy's and St Thomas' NHS Foundation Trust, London, UK

Neil S. Sheerin
Professor of Renal Medicine, Newcastle University and Medical School, Newcastle, UK

John Taylor
Consultant Transplant Surgeon, Guy's and St Thomas' NHS Foundation Trust, London, UK

Judy Taylor
Consultant Paediatric Nephrologist, Evelina Children's Hospital, Guy's and St Thomas' NHS Foundation Trust, London, UK

Katie Vinen
Consultant Nephrologist, King's College Hospital NHS Foundation Trust, London, UK

Hayley Wells
Chief Renal Pharmacist, Guy's and St Thomas' NHS Foundation Trust, London, UK

Eleri Wood
Senior Sister Low Clearance & Transplant Clinics, King's College Hospital NHS Foundation Trust, London, UK

Preface

This is the second edition of this popular handbook on kidney disease. It is necessary because important advances have been made in several areas, including the treatment of the anaemia associated with chronic kidney disease. Moreover, with the passage of time, more is now known about the prevalence, and importance, of chronic kidney disease in the United Kingdom and the rest of the world. In this second edition, we refine the presentation of the information concerning chronic kidney disease, we expand on the importance of good preparation for dialysis and transplantation, where those options are relevant, and we expand on the important area of conservative, or non-dialytic, management of the symptoms of chronic kidney disease, an option which is taken by increasing numbers. We have also revised the appendices, which include a Top Ten Tips section for quick reference. All in all, we hope and feel that this new version is an improvement on its predecessor, and that readers (from students to non-kidney specialists) will find this book a useful guide to the best management of a growing number of patients.

CHAPTER 1

Diagnostic Tests in Chronic Kidney Disease

Behdad Afzali[1], Satish Jayawardene[2] and David Goldsmith[1]

[1]King's College London, London, UK
[2]King's College Hospital NHS Foundation Trust, London, UK

OVERVIEW

- Urinary protein excretion of <150 mg/day is normal (~30 mg of this is albumin and about 70–100 mg is Tamm-Horsfall (muco)protein, derived from the proximal renal tubule). Protein excretion can rise transiently with fever, acute illness, urinary tract infection (UTI) and orthostatically. In pregnancy, the upper limit of normal protein excretion is around 300 mg/day. Persistent elevation of albumin excretion (microalbuminuria) and other proteins can indicate renal or systemic illness.

- Repeat positive dipstick tests for blood and protein in the urine two or three times to ensure the findings are persistent.

- Microalbuminuria is an early sign of renal and cardiovascular dysfunction with adverse prognostic significance.

- Non-visible haematuria (NVH) is present in around 4% of the adult population – of whom at least 50% have glomerular disease.

- If initial glomerular filtration rate (GFR) is normal, and proteinuria is absent, progressive loss of GFR amongst those people with NVH of renal origin is rare, although long-term (and usually community-based) follow-up is still recommended.

- Adults aged 40 years old or more should undergo cystoscopy if they have NVH.

- Any patient with NVH who has abnormal renal function, proteinuria, hypertension and a normal cystoscopy should be referred to a nephrologist.

- Blood pressure control, reduction of proteinuria and cholesterol reduction are all useful therapeutic manoeuvres in those with renal causes of NVH.

- All NVH patients should have long-term follow-up of their renal function and blood pressure (this can, and often should be, community-based).

- Renal function is measured using creatinine, and this is now routinely converted into an estimated glomerular filtration rate (eGFR) value quickly and easily.

- The most common imaging technique now used for the kidney is the renal ultrasound, which can detect size, shape, symmetry of kidneys and presence of tumour, stone or renal obstruction.

Symptoms of chronic kidney disease (CKD) are often non-specific (Table 1.1). Clinical signs (of CKD, or of systemic diseases or syndromes) may be present and recognized early on in the natural history of kidney disease but, more often, both symptoms and signs are only present and recognized very late – sometimes too late to permit effective treatment in time to prepare for dialysis. However, the most commonly performed test of renal function – plasma creatinine – is typically performed with every hospital inpatient and as part of investigations or screening during many GP surgery or hospital clinic outpatient episodes.

Unlike 'angina' or 'chronic obstructive airways disease', where a history can be revealing (e.g. walking distance or cough), there is little that is quantifiable about CKD severity without blood and/or urine testing.

This is why serendipitous discovery of kidney problems (haematuria, proteinuria, structural abnormalities on kidney imaging or loss of kidney function) is a common 'presentation'. A full understanding of what these abnormalities mean and a clear guide to 'what to do next' are particularly needed in kidney medicine, and filling this gap is one of the aims of this book.

Correct use and interpretation of urine dipsticks and plasma creatinine values (by far the commonest tests used for screening and identification of kidney disease) is the main focus of this chapter. Renal imaging and renal biopsy will also be described briefly.

Urine testing

Urinalysis is a basic test for the presence and severity of kidney disease. Testing urine during the menstrual period in women, and within 2–3 days of heavy strenuous exercise in both genders, should

Table 1.1 Signs and symptoms of chronic kidney disease.

Symptoms	Signs
Tiredness	Pallor
Anorexia	Leuconychia
Nausea and vomiting	Peripheral oedema
Itching	Pleural effusion
Nocturia, frequency, oliguria	Pulmonary oedema
Haematuria	Raised blood pressure
Frothy urine	
Loin pain	

ABC of Kidney Disease, Second edition.
Edited by David Goldsmith, Satish Jayawardene and Penny Ackland.
© 2013 John Wiley & Sons, Ltd. Published 2013 by John Wiley & Sons, Ltd.

be avoided, to avoid contamination or artefacts. Fresh 'mid-stream' urine is best, again to reduce accidental contamination. Refrigeration of urine at temperatures from +2 to +8°C assists preservation. Specimens that have languished in an overstretched hospital laboratory specimen reception area, before eventually undergoing analysis, will rarely reveal all of the potential information that could have been gained.

Changes in urine colour are usually noticed by patients. Table 1.2 shows the main causes of different-coloured urine. Chemical parameters of the urine that can be detected using dipsticks include urine pH, haemoglobin, glucose, protein, leucocyte esterase, nitrites and ketones. Figure 1.1 shows the dipstick in its 'dry' state and an example of a positive test. Table 1.3 shows the main false negative and false positive results that can interfere with correct interpretation.

Urine microscopy can only add useful information to urinalysis when there is a reliable methodology for collection, storage and

Table 1.3 The main causes of false negative and false positive testing from use of urine dipsticks.

Test	False positive	False negative
Haemoglobin	Myoglobin Microbial peroxidases	Ascorbic acid Delayed examination
Proteinuria	Very alkaline urine (pH 9) Chlorhexidine	Tubular proteins Immunoglobulin light chains Globulins
Glucose	Oxidizing detergents	UTI Ascorbic acid

Discounting contamination from menstrual – or other – bleeding, and exercise-induced haematuria and proteinuria.

analysis. This is often lacking, even in hospitals. Early-morning urine is best, with rapid sample centrifugation. Under ideal circumstances *cells* (erythrocytes, leucocytes, renal tubular cells and urinary epithelial cells), *casts* (cylinders of proteinaceous matrix), *crystals, lipids* and *organisms* can be reliably identified where present in urine. Figure 1.2 shows a red cell cast in urine (indicative of acute renal inflammation). Figure 1.3 shows urinary crystals.

Table 1.2 The main causes of differently coloured urine.

Pink–red–brown–black	Yellow–brown	Blue–green
Gross haematuria (e.g. bladder or renal tumour; IgA nephropathy)	**Jaundice** **Drugs:**	**Drugs:** triamterene
Haemoglobinuria (e.g. drug reaction)	chloroquine, nitrofurantoin	**Dyes:** methylene blue
Myoglobinuria (e.g. rhabdomyolysis)		
Acute intermittent porphyria		
Alkaptonuria		
Drugs: phenytoin, rifampicin (red); metronidazole, methyldopa (darkening on standing)		
Foods: beetroot, blackberries		

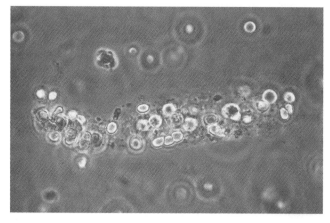

Figure 1.2 Microscopy of centrifuged fresh urine. There is a red cell cast (protein skeleton with incorporated red blood cells). This is characteristic of acute glomerulonephritis.

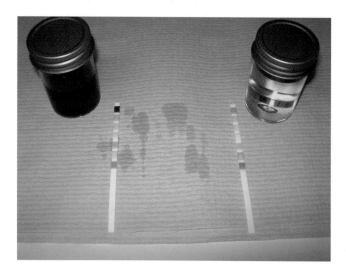

Figure 1.1 Urine dipstick – the urine on the right is normal and the colours of all of the squares on the urine dipstick are normal/negative. The urine on the left is from someone with acute glomerulonephritis, looks pink-brown macroscopically and has maximal blood and protein on the dipstick.

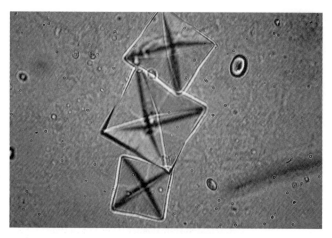

Figure 1.3 Crystalluria.

Non-visible haematuria

Definition and background

In healthy people red blood cells (rbc) are not present in the urine in > 95% of cases. Large numbers of rbcs make the urine pink or red.

Non-visible haematuria (NVH) (formerly known as microscopic haematuria) is commonly defined as the presence of greater than two rbcs per high power field in a centrifuged urine sediment. It is seen in 3–6% of the normal population, and in 5–10% of those relatives of kidney patients who undergo screening for potential kidney donation.

NVH can be an incidental finding of no prognostic importance, or the first sign of intrinsic renal disease or urological malignancy. It always requires assessment, and most often requires referral to a kidney specialist or to a urologist.

Clinical features

The finding of NVH is usually as a result of routine medical examination for employment, insurance or GP-registration purposes in an otherwise apparently healthy adult. Initially, therefore, NVH is an issue for primary healthcare workers. The goal of an assessment is to understand whether:

- there are any clues available from the patient's history, his/her family history or from examination to point to a particular diagnosis, e.g. connective tissue disease, sickle cell disease;
- the haematuria is transient or persistent;
- there is any evidence of renal disease, e.g. abnormal renal function, accompanying proteinuria, raised blood pressure (BP);
- the haematuria represents glomerular (i.e. from the kidney) or extra-glomerular (urological) bleeding.

Investigations

Typically, the full evaluation of NVH requires hospital-based investigations. Box 1.1 lists these in a logical order.

Box 1.1 Investigations required for the work-up of patients with non-visible haematuria

- Protein:creatinine ratio on fresh urine (if present on urinary dipstick testing)
- Urine microscopy and culture
- Plasma biochemistry and eGFR
- Autoantibody screen, e.g. antinuclear antibody (ANA) and antineutrophil cytoplasmic antibody (ANCA) and complement levels (C3 and C4)
- Renal ultrasound
- Renal CT/MRI (in certain cases)
- Cystoscopy for adults > 40 years of age
- Renal biopsy in certain circumstances

- *Urine microscopy and culture* should also be undertaken. The presence of dysmorphic red cells in the urine increases the possibility of intrinsic/parenchymal kidney disease as opposed to urological disease. This can only be ascertained in a specialist laboratory.

- *Renal structure* can be assessed with a renal ultrasound scan (this can show stones, cysts and tumours). A plain abdominal film will show radio-opaque renal, ureteric or bladder calculi. Renal function should be assessed by measurement of plasma biochemistry and estimated glomerular filtration rate (eGFR). In addition, proteinuria should be looked for by dipstick analysis of the urine and, if present, a protein/creatinine ratio measured. Proteinuria > 0.5 g/24 h (protein:creatinine ratio > 50) suggests glomerular disease and a referral to a kidney specialist is warranted for NVH with significant proteinuria, raised BP or abnormal renal function.

Management

Any patient who presents with persistent non-visible haematuria over the age of 40 should be referred to a urologist. A renal ultrasound, urine cytology and a flexible cystoscopy to exclude urological cancer would normally be undertaken.

Any patient who has abnormal renal function, proteinuria, hypertension and a normal cystoscopy should be referred to a kidney specialist.

Renal biopsy is required to establish a diagnosis with absolute certainty in most cases of 'renal haematuria'. Those patients who additionally have renal impairment, heavy proteinuria, hypertension, positive autoantibodies, low complement levels or have a family history of renal disease should be considered for a renal biopsy.

Please also see the 2008 NICE CKD guidelines for further information on NVH, http://www.nice.org.uk/nicemedia/live/12069/42119/42119.pdf.

Prognosis

The prognosis for most patients with asymptomatic NVH without urological malignancy and no evidence of intrinsic renal disease is very good. It is beyond the scope of this chapter to discuss the prognosis of all the causes of non-visible haematuria, as listed in Table 1.4. However, some general observations apply for those patients in whom there is no structural cause for NVH and bleeding is glomerular, and these are given below.

In the presence of impaired renal function, it is mandatory to try to achieve blood pressure control (<130/80 mmHg) and reduction of microalbuminuria or proteinuria (if present). Angiotensin converting enzyme (ACE) inhibitors or angiotensin II receptor blockers (ARBs) are useful agents, as they achieve both of these desired effects. It is very important to recheck plasma creatinine and potassium about 7–14 days after starting ACE or ARB, and regularly thereafter – an increase of $\geq$ 30% in plasma creatinine or a fall of $\geq$ 25% eGFR, or a rise of plasma potassium to exceed 5.5 mmol/L, should occasion recall to consider abandoning the drugs or reducing the dose, further investigations, and dietary advice for potassium restriction if relevant.

It is important that these patients, whether monitored in the community or at a hospital-based clinic, have their urine tested, BP measured and renal function monitored regularly. If not under renal specialist follow-up, the development of hypertension, proteinuria or deterioration in renal function are all indications for referral to a specialist unit (see Chapter 3).

Table 1.4 Causes of non-visible haematuria.

Renal causes	Systemic causes	Miscellaneous and urological causes
IgA nephropathy	Systemic lupus erythematosus	Cystic diseases of the kidney
Thin basement membrane disease	Henoch–Schönlein purpura	Papillary necrosis
Alport's syndrome		Urothelial tumours
Focal segmental glomerulosclerosis		Renal and bladder stones
Membranoproliferative glomerulonephritis		Exercise-induced haematuria
Post-infectious glomerulonephritis		

Microalbuminuria and proteinuria

Protein is normally present in urine in small quantities. Tubular proteins (e.g. Tamm-Horsfall) and low amounts of albumin can be detected in healthy people. Microalbuminuria (MAU) refers to the presence of elevated urinary albumin concentrations (see Table 1.5); MAU is a sign of either systemic or renal malfunction.

MAU is measured by quantitative immunoassay – and is an important first and early sign of many renal conditions, particularly diabetic renal disease and other glomerulopathies. It is also strongly associated with adverse cardiovascular outcomes. Around 10% of the population can be shown to have persistent MAU. For confirmation, two out of three consecutive analyses should show MAU in the same three-month period.

UAER (urinary albumin excretion rate) – in a healthy population the normal range for UAER is 1.5–20 µg/min. UAER increases with strenuous exercise, a high-protein diet, pregnancy and urinary tract infections (UTIs). Daytime UAER is 25% higher than at night (so for daytime urine, an upper normal limit of 30 µg/min is often used). Overnight timed collections can be performed (and microalbuminuric range is an overnight UAER of 20–200 µg/min), but for unselected population screening the albumin:creatinine ratio (ACR) in early-morning urine is preferable. An ACR of > 2 predicts a UAER of > 30 µg/min with a high sensitivity.

Increasingly favoured as a screening tool is the urinary protein:creatinine ratio (**PCR**). This is best done on 'spot' early-morning urine samples (as renal protein excretion has a diurnal rhythm; see below). This is now preferable to relying on 24-hour urine collections. There is an inherent assumption in using PCR that urinary creatinine concentration is 10 mmol/L (in practice it can range from 2 to 30), but this is of little practical importance for its use as a screening tool. A PCR of 100 mg/mmol corresponds roughly to 1 g/L of proteinuria.

One question often asked is how to 'convert' an ACR to a PCR. At low levels of proteinuria (<1 g/day), a rough conversion is that doubling the ACR will give you the PCR. At proteinuria excretion rates of > 1 g/day, the relationship is more accurately represented by $1.3 \times ACR = PCR$.

Table 1.5 attempts to display all of the different ways to express urinary protein to allow for comparisons between methods.

Please note that the normal range for protein excretion in pregnancy is up to 300 mg/day, with clinical significance (pre-eclampsia or renal disease) being more likely once 500 mg or more is excreted per day. See Chapter 6.

Please also see the 2008 NICE CKD guidelines on albuminuria, proteinuria and eGFR, http://www.nice.org.uk/nicemedia/live/12069/42119/42119.pdf.

Tests of kidney function

The kidney has exocrine and endocrine functions. The most important function to assess, however, is renal excretory capacity, which we measure as glomerular filtration rate (GFR). Each kidney has about 1 million nephrons, and the measured GFR is the composite function of all nephrons in both kidneys. Conceptually, it can be understood as the (virtual) clearance of a substance from a volume of plasma into the urine per unit of time. The substance can be endogenous (creatinine, cystatin C) or exogenous (inulin, iohexol, iothalamate, ^{51}Cr-EDTA, ^{99m}Tc-DTPA). This 'ideal substance' to measure kidney function does not exist – ideal characteristics being free filtration across the glomerulus, neither reabsorption from nor excretion into renal tubules, existing in a steady state concentration in plasma, and being easily and reliably measured. Despite creatinine failing several of these criteria, it is universally used, and we shall concentrate on interpreting creatinine concentration in urine and blood as it aids derivation of GFR.

The basic anatomy of the kidney and the anatomy and basic physiology of the 'nephron' (the functional component of the kidney), are shown in Figure 7.1.

Table 1.6 shows the different ways in which both plasma urea and plasma creatinine may be 'artefactually' elevated or reduced, which can lead to misunderstanding and miscalculation of renal

Table 1.5 Equivalent ranges for urinary protein loss.

	Urine dipstick	Albumin excretion rate (AER) (µg/min; mg/24 h)		Urinary albumin:creatinine ratio (mg/mmol)	Protein (mg)/ creatinine (mmol)	Urinary protein (mg/24 h)
Normal	0	6–20	10–30	<2.5 (m) <3.5 (w)	<15	<150
Microalbuminuria	0	>20–200	30–300	>2.5 (m) >3.5 (w)	<15	<150
'Trace' proteinuria	Trace	>200	>300	15–29	15–29	150–299
Proteinuria	+, ++	N/A	N/A	N/A	30–350	300–3500
Nephrotic	+++	N/A	N/A	N/A	>350	>3.5 g

m, men; w, women.

Table 1.6 Problems with sole reliance on plasma concentrations of urea and creatinine to determine renal function.

Factors independent of renal function that can affect plasma urea	Factors independent of renal function that can affect plasma creatinine	Other factors that can affect interpretation of plasma creatinine values
Hydration	Diet (meat)	Use of Jaffe reaction in laboratories: interference by glucose, ascorbate, acetoacetate
Burns	Creatine supplements (e.g. body builders)	
Steroids	Age	Use of enzymatic reaction in laboratories: interference by ethamsylate or flucytosine
Diuretics	Body habitus	
Liver disease	Race	
Diet (protein)		

function. Creatinine is measured by two quite different techniques in the laboratory – one, the Jaffe reaction, relies on creatinine reacting with an alkaline picrate solution but is not specific for creatinine (e.g. cephalosporins, acetoacetate and ascorbate), while the other, the enzymatic method, is more accurate. Eventually, isotope-dilution mass spectroscopy (IDMS) may render both of these variously flawed techniques redundant, either by direct substitution of method or by allowing IDMS-traceable creatinine values to be reported.

Creatinine is produced at an almost constant rate from muscle-derived creatine and phosphocreatine. However, as can be seen from Figure 1.4, it is an insensitive marker of early loss of renal function (fall in GFR), and as renal function declines there is correspondingly more tubular creatinine secretion. It varies with diet, gender, disease state and muscle mass.

Estimated glomerular filtration rate

The manipulation of plasma creatinine to derive a rapid estimation of creatinine clearance is very useful clinically, and is now formally recommended (as of April 2006 – see Chapters 3 and 4) to aid appropriate identification and referral of patients with CKD. There are several formulaic ways of doing this, and the formula that has been adopted in the United Kingdom, United States and many countries is the four-variable Modification Diet in Renal Disease (MDRD) equation (Figure 1.5 and Chapter 3), but it

must be appreciated that this formula has not been validated in ethnic minority patients, in older patients, in pregnant women, the malnourished, amputees or in children under 16 years of age.

Useful though deriving a value for GFR is, the value derived using the MDRD formula is only an *estimate* whose accuracy diminishes as GFR exceeds 60 mL/min, and values should therefore be viewed as having significant error margins rather than being precise. Values can only properly be used when renal function is in 'steady state', i.e. not in acute kidney injury. It is unwise to rely exclusively on the formula when the eGFR is between 60 and 89 mL/min (CKD stage 2), because of its shortcomings, while values > 90 mL/min should be reported thus (i.e. not as a precise figure). There is an urgent unmet need for better markers, and better formulae.

Formal nuclear medicine or research-laboratory-derived measures of GFR are expensive, time-consuming and largely (and increasingly) confined to research studies.

Please also see the 2008 NICE CKD guidelines for the assessment and interpretation of kidney function/eGFR, http://www.nice.org.uk/nicemedia/live/12069/42119/42119.pdf.

Renal imaging

There is a wide range of imaging techniques available to localize and interrogate the kidneys. Table 1.7 gives the preferred methods for a range of conditions. Intravascular contrast studies are still used, though ultrasound has replaced most IVU/IVP

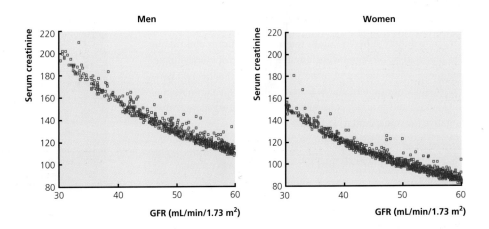

Figure 1.4 Relationship between plasma creatinine and glomerular filtration rate.

$$\text{GFR (mL/min/1.73 m}^2) = 175 \times [\text{serum creatinine (μmol/L)} \times 0.011312] - 1.154 \times [\text{age}] - 0.203 \times [1.212 \text{ if black}] \times [0.742 \text{ if female}]$$

Figure 1.5 Four-variable Modification Diet in Renal Disease equation for estimated glomerular filtration rate.

Table 1.7 Renal imaging techniques and their main indications/applications.

Condition	Technique
Renal failure	Ultrasound
Proteinuria/nephrotic syndrome	Ultrasound
Renal artery stenosis	MRA
Renal stones	Plain abdominal film
	Non-contrast CT
Renal infection	Ultrasound or CT abdomen
Retroperitoneal fibrosis	CT abdomen

MRA, magnetic resonance angiogram.

(Intravenous urogram/intravenous pyelogram) examinations. Low osmolar non-ionic agents are less nephrotoxic and better tolerated. Reactions to contrast agents can be severe, though rarely life-threatening. In addition, renal impairment (usually mild and reversible, sometimes severe and irreversible) can be seen after the use of intravenous contrast. In patients with a plasma creatinine > 130 µmol/L (eGFR <60 mL/min), thought must be given to the wisdom of the investigation. Pre-existing renal impairment, advanced age, diabetes and diuretic use or dehydration significantly increase the risk of contrast-induced nephropathy. The mainstay of prevention is understanding the risk and avoiding dehydration (by judiciously hydrating patients and promoting urine flow) using saline or 0.45% sodium bicarbonate. The dopamine agonist fenoldopam and the antioxidant *N*-acetylcysteine have both been proposed as protective agents; oral *N*-acetylcysteine has been widely assessed with conflicting results and its role remains uncertain. However, it is an inexpensive agent without significant side-effects, and its use in clinical practice may not therefore be inappropriate.

A comprehensive review of all imaging techniques is beyond the scope of this chapter. We shall concentrate on *ultrasound* imaging as this is by far the most often used for screening and investigation. Reference to radionuclide imaging and IVU/IVP is made in Chapter 12. Renal size is usually in proportion to body height, and normally lies between 9 and 12 cm. Box 1.2 shows reasons for enlarged or shrunken kidneys. The *echo-consistency* of the renal cortex is reduced compared to medulla and the collecting system. In adults the loss of this 'corticomedullary differentiation' is a sensitive but non-specific marker of CKD. Apart from renal size and corticomedullary differentiation, the other significant abnormalities reported by ultrasound include the presence of cysts (simple, complex), solid lesions and urinary obstruction. Figure 1.6 shows a normal kidney (a) and an obstructed kidney (b). Examination of the bladder and prostate is usually undertaken alongside scanning of native (or transplanted) kidneys.

Box 1.2 **Reasons for enlarged or shrunken kidneys on renal imaging**

Large kidneys – symmetrical
Diabetes
Acromegaly
Amyloidosis
Lymphoma

Large kidney – asymmetrical
Compensatory hypertrophy (e.g. secondary to nephrectomy)
Renal vein thrombosis

Large kidneys – irregular outline
Polycystic kidney disease
Other multicystic disease

Small kidneys – symmetrical
Chronic kidney disease
Bilateral renal artery stenosis
Bilateral hypoplasia

Small kidney – unilateral
Renal artery stenosis
Unilateral hypoplasia
Scarring from reflux nephropathy

Renal angiography and other techniques relevant to renal blood vessels are covered in Chapter 8. Radionuclide imaging is used for renal scars and urinary reflux, which is also mentioned in part in Chapter 12.

Renal biopsy

A renal biopsy is undertaken to investigate and diagnose renal disease in native and transplanted kidneys. Table 1.8 shows the main indications, contra-indications and complications of this

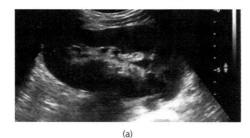

(a)

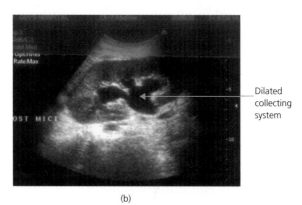

Dilated collecting system

(b)

Figure 1.6 (a) Ultrasound appearance of a normal kidney: dark areas represent renal cortex, and the central white area is the renal pelvis and collecting system. (b) An obstructed kidney, which shows in its centre a severely dilated renal pelvis and calyces (containing urine which is 'dark' on ultrasound).

Table 1.8 Indications for renal biopsy.

Indications	Contraindications	Complications
Nephrotic syndrome	Multiple renal cysts	Pain
Systemic disease with proteinuria or kidney failure	Solitary kidney (relative)	Bleeding – haematoma, haematuria (significant in <5%)
Acute kidney injury	Acute pyelonephritis/abscess	Other organ biopsied (e.g. colon, spleen, liver)
Proteinuria (PCR > 50–100)	Renal neoplasm	Arteriovenous fistula (0.1%)
Proteinuria and micro/macro-haematuria	Uncontrolled blood pressure	Nephrectomy (<0.1%)
Unexplained chronic kidney disease	Abnormal blood clotting	Death (<0.01%)
Transplanted kidney	Morbid obesity (relative) Inability to consent to, or to comply with instructions	

PCR: protein:creatinine ratio.

test. It is a highly specialized investigation, which should only be performed after careful consideration of the risk/benefit ratio, and with the close support of experienced imaging and renal histopathological teams.

Further reading

Fink HA, Ishani A, Taylor BC, Greer NL, MacDonald R, Rossini D, Sadiq S, Lankireddy S, Kane RL, Wilt TJ (2012) Screening for, monitoring, and treatment of chronic kidney disease stages 1 to 3: a systematic review for the U.S. Preventive Services Task Force and for an American College of Physicians Clinical Practice Guideline. *Ann Intern Med* **156**(8):570–81.

Maione A, Navaneethan SD, Graziano G, Mitchell R, Johnson D, Mann JF, Gao P, Craig JC, Tognoni G, Perkovic V, Nicolucci A, De Cosmo S, Sasso A, Lamacchia O, Cignarelli M, Manfreda VM, Gentile G, Strippoli GF (2011) Angiotensin-converting enzyme inhibitors, angiotensin receptor blockers and combined therapy in patients with micro- and macroalbuminuria and other cardiovascular risk factors: a systematic review of randomized controlled trials. *Nephrol Dial Transplant* **26**(9):2827–47.

NHS Evidence: http://www.evidence.nhs.uk/topic/kidney-failure

Redon J, Martinez F (2012) Microalbuminuria as surrogate endpoint in therapeutic trials. *Curr Hypertens Rep* **14**(4):345–9.

Van de Wal RM, Voors AA, Gansevoort RT (2006) Urinary albumin excretion and the renin-angiotensin system in cardiovascular risk management. *Expert Opin Pharmacother* **7**(18): 2505–20.

www.renal.org/eGFR/haematuria.html

www.renal.org/eGFR/proteinuria.html

www.renal.org/eGFR/refer.html

http://www.nice.org.uk/nicemedia/live/12069/42119/42119.pdf

CHAPTER 2

Acute Kidney Injury (Formerly Known as Acute Renal Failure)

Rachel Hilton

Guy's and St Thomas' NHS Foundation Trust, London, UK

OVERVIEW

- The term acute kidney injury (AKI) is now preferred in kidney circles to the older term acute renal failure (ARF).

- The life-threatening consequences of AKI are volume overload, hyperkalaemia and metabolic acidosis.

- AKI is more common in older patients and those with underlying chronic kidney disease (CKD).

- Precipitating factors include hypovolaemia and hypotension (pre-renal); the use of nephrotoxic drugs and radiographic contrast (intrinsic renal); and obstruction from e.g. stones, malignancy or retroperitoneal fibrosis (post-renal).

- Prevention strategies include maintaining adequate blood pressure (BP), ensuring adequate volume status and avoiding potentially nephrotoxic drugs.

- AKI is frequently reversible, and rapid recognition and treatment may prevent irreversible nephron loss.

- If past creatinine measurements are not available, useful differentiating features of acute (as opposed to chronic) renal failure may be the absence of anaemia, hypocalcaemia, hyperphosphataemia and/or reduced renal size and cortical thickness, which often accompany CKD.

- Acute tubular necrosis (ATN) is the commonest cause of intrinsic renal disease, and if the precipitating factor has been removed or treated, prognosis is generally good. However, other causes must always be excluded as they have important management implications:
  - rashes, arthralgia or myalgia may suggest an underlying multisystem disease;
  - antibiotics or nonsteroidal anti-inflammatory drugs NSAIDs may cause interstitial nephritis;
  - non-visible haematuria or proteinuria, or dysmorphic red cells or red cell casts, may suggest renal inflammation such as glomerulonephritis or acute interstitial nephritis.

Definition and classification

Acute kidney injury (AKI) is characterized in an abrupt fall in glomerular filtration rate (GFR), clinically manifest as an abrupt

ABC of Kidney Disease, Second edition.
Edited by David Goldsmith, Satish Jayawardene and Penny Ackland.
© 2013 John Wiley & Sons, Ltd. Published 2013 by John Wiley & Sons, Ltd.

and sustained rise in urea and creatinine. Potentially life threatening consequences include volume overload, hyperkalaemia and metabolic acidosis. The RIFLE criteria classify AKI according to degree and outcome (Figure 2.1). A revised definition of AKI based upon modifications to the RIFLE and Acute Kidney Injury Network (AKIN) criteria has been made by the KDIGO clinical practice guidelines (Table 2.1).

Epidemiology

AKI is increasingly common: this probably reflects true increased incidence, and better detection. Recent data suggest an incidence of AKI, defined as serum creatinine above $500\,\mu\,mol/L$, of around 500 per million population (pmp) per year, which is twice the UK prevalence of haemodialysis patients and therefore places high demands upon healthcare resources. AKI is more common with increasing age, the highest incidence being in the 80- to 89-year-old age group (950 pmp/year).

AKI (as per KDIGO criteria) complicates at least 20% of emergency hospital admissions, mostly in patients with underlying chronic kidney disease (CKD), and is generally multifactorial in nature chiefly associated with hypovolaemia, hypotension and the use of nephrotoxic drugs or radiographic contrast. When severe enough to require dialysis, in-hospital mortality is around 50%, and may exceed 75% in the context of sepsis or in the critically ill.

Aetiology

The causes of AKI can be grouped into three major categories (Figure 2.2):

- decreased renal blood flow (pre-renal; 40–80% of cases);
- direct renal parenchymal damage (intrinsic renal; 35–40% of cases);
- obstructed urine flow (post-renal or obstructive; 2–10% of cases).

Pre-renal acute kidney injury

Renal blood flow (RBF) and GFR remain roughly constant over a wide range of mean arterial pressures owing to changes in afferent (pre-glomerular) and efferent (post-glomerular) arteriolar resistance. Below 70 mmHg, autoregulation is impaired

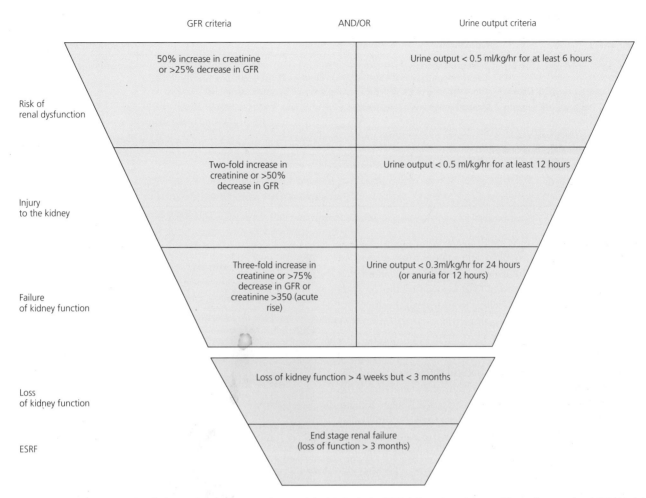

Figure 2.1 Acute kidney injury classified according to degree and outcome by RIFLE criteria. RIFLE defines three degrees of increasing severity of AKI (risk, injury and failure) and two possible outcomes (loss and ESRF).

Table 2.1 AKI classified according to serum creatinine and urine output criteria. The diagnostic criteria for AKI are an abrupt (within 48 hours) absolute increase in the serum creatinine concentration of ≥ 0.3 mg/dL (26.4 μmol/L) from baseline, a percentage increase in the serum creatinine concentration of $\geq 50\%$, or oliguria of less than 0.5 mL/kg per hour for more than six hours.

Stage	Serum creatinine criteria	Urine output criteria
1	Increase in serum creatinine of more than or equal to 0.3 mg/dL (≥ 26.4 μmol/L) or increase to more than or equal to 150 to 200% (1.5- to 2-fold) from baseline	Less than 0.5 mL/kg per hour for more than 6 hours
2	Increase in serum creatinine to more than 200 to 300% (> 2- to 3-fold) from baseline	Less than 0.5 mL/kg per hour for more than 12 hours
3	Increase in serum creatinine to more than 300% (> 3-fold) from baseline (or serum creatinine of more than or equal to 4.0 mg/dL [≥ 354 μmol/L] with an acute increase of at least 0.5 mg/dL [44 μmol/L])	Less than 0.3 mL/kg per hour for 24 hours or anuria for 12 hours

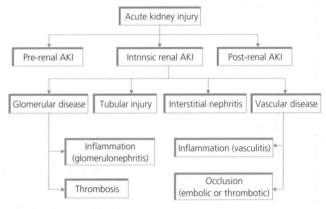

Figure 2.2 Aetiology: acute kidney injury.

vasoconstriction mediated by angiotensin II. Drugs that interfere with these mediators may provoke pre-renal AKI (Table 2.2) in certain settings. With renal artery stenosis or volume depletion, GFR maintenance is particularly angiotensin II-dependent. Use of angiotensin converting enzyme (ACE) inhibitors or angiotensin II receptor antagonists can induce AKI. With volume depletion, angiotensin II and noradrenaline levels are generally high, and in

and GFR falls proportionately. Renal autoregulation chiefly depends on a combination of afferent arteriolar vasodilatation mediated by prostaglandins and nitric oxide, and efferent arteriolar

Table 2.2 Principal causes of pre-renal acute kidney injury.

Hypovolaemia	Hypotension	Renal hypoperfusion	Oedema states
Haemorrhage	Cardiogenic shock	Reduced renal perfusion plus impaired autoregulation (e.g. hypovolaemia plus NSAID/COX2 inhibitor or ACE inhibitor/angiotensin II receptor antagonist)	Cardiac failure
GI losses (e.g. vomiting, diarrhoea)	Distributive shock (e.g. sepsis, anaphylaxis)	Abdominal aortic aneurysm	Hepatic cirrhosis
Urinary losses (e.g. glycosuria, post-obstructive diuresis, diuretics)		Renal artery stenosis/occlusion	Nephrotic syndrome (particularly minimal change nephropathy)
Cutaneous losses (e.g. burns)		Hepatorenal syndrome	
Fluid redistribution (e.g. GI obstruction, pancreatitis)			

GI, gastrointestinal; NSAID, nonsteroidal anti-inflammatory drug; COX2, Cyclooxygenase; ACE, angiotensin converting enzyme.

this setting NSAIDs (nonsteroidal anti-inflammatory drugs) or cyclooxygenase (COX) inhibitors, which inhibit prostaglandin synthesis, permit unopposed action of local vasoconstrictors on both afferent and efferent arterioles, leading to an acute decline in GFR.

Intrinsic renal acute kidney injury

Parenchymal causes of AKI may be subdivided into those primarily affecting the glomeruli, the tubules, the intrarenal vasculature or the renal interstitium. Overall, the commonest cause is acute tubular necrosis (ATN) (Figures 2.3 and 2.4), resulting from continuation of the same pathophysiological processes that lead to pre-renal hypoperfusion. In intensive care, the commonest cause is sepsis, frequently accompanied by multi-organ failure. Post-operative ATN accounts for up to 25% of cases of hospital-acquired AKI, mostly due to pre-renal causes. The third commonest cause of hospital-acquired AKI is acute radiocontrast nephropathy. See also Table 2.3.

Post-renal acute kidney injury

Obstructive nephropathy presents as AKI relatively infrequently, but rapid diagnosis by ultrasound and prompt intervention to relieve obstruction can result in improvement or even complete

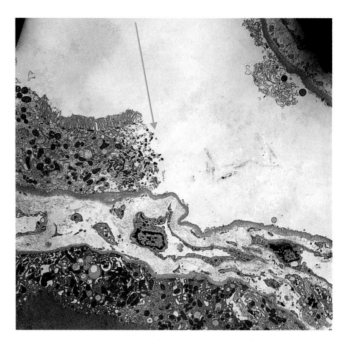

Figure 2.4 Electron micrograph of disrupted renal tubular epithelium in acute tubular necrosis. The arrow points to the segment where the delicate microvillous tubular epithelial lining is lost.

recovery of renal function. An important clinical consequence is the substantial diuresis that generally occurs once obstruction is relieved, which requires careful monitoring and appropriate fluid replacement to avoid volume depletion. See also Table 2.4.

Prevention

The key preventative strategy is to identify patients most at risk, including older patients, those with diabetes, hypertension or vascular disease and patients with pre-existing renal impairment. Appropriate preventative measures include maintenance of adequate blood pressure (BP) and volume status and avoidance of potentially nephrotoxic agents, particularly NSAIDs, ACE inhibitors or angiotensin II receptor blockers (ARB), as discussed earlier. Among the many causes of AKI, radiocontrast nephropathy is potentially preventable. In high-risk patients, radiocontrast procedures should be limited where possible and alternative imaging considered.

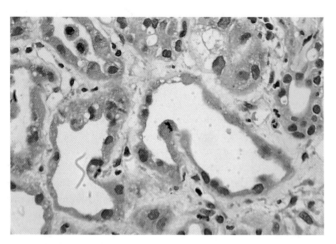

Figure 2.3 A histological view of renal tubular dilatation and loss of renal tubular epithelial cells in acute kidney injury ('acute tubular necrosis').

Table 2.3 Principal causes of intrinsic renal acute kidney injury.

Glomerular disease	Tubular injury	Interstitial nephritis	Vascular
Inflammatory: e.g. post-infectious glomerulonephritis, cryoglobulinaemia, Henoch–Schönlein purpura, SLE, ANCA-associated glomerulonephritis, anti-GBM disease	Ischaemia: prolonged renal hypoperfusion	Drug-induced: e.g. NSAIDs, antibiotics	Vasculitis (usually ANCA-associated)
Thrombotic: e.g. DIC (Figure 2.5), thrombotic microangiopathy	Toxins: drugs (e.g. aminoglycosides), radiocontrast, pigments (e.g. myoglobin), heavy metals (e.g. cisplatinum)	Infiltrative: e.g. lymphoma	Cryoglobulinaemia
	Metabolic: hypercalcaemia, immunoglobulin light chains	Granulomatous: sarcoidosis, TB	Polyarteritis nodosa
	Crystals: e.g. urate, oxalate	Infection-related: e.g. post-infective; pyelonephritis	Thrombotic microangiopathy
			Cholesterol emboli
			Renal artery or renal vein thrombosis

SLE, systemic lupus erythematosus; ANCA, antineutrophil cytoplasmic antibody; GBM, glomerular basement membrane; DIC, disseminated intravascular coagulation; NSAIDs, nonsteroidal anti-inflammatory drugs; TB, tuberculosis.

Table 2.4 Principal causes of post-renal acute kidney injury.

Intrinsic	Extrinsic
Intraluminal: e.g. stone, blood clot, papillary necrosis	Pelvic malignancy
Intramural: e.g. urethral stricture, prostatic hypertrophy or malignancy, bladder tumour, radiation fibrosis	Retroperitoneal fibrosis

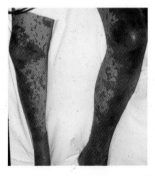

Figure 2.5 Disseminated intravascular coagulation (DIC).

Intravascular volume depletion is a key risk factor, which can be corrected by appropriate volume expansion with intravenous saline. Oral use of the antioxidant *N*-acetylcysteine has been widely assessed with conflicting results, and its role remains uncertain. However, it is an inexpensive agent without significant side-effects and its use in clinical practice may therefore be appropriate.

Differential diagnosis

AKI is frequently reversible, and rapid recognition and treatment may prevent irreversible nephron loss. The diagnostic approach to the patient with AKI involves a careful history, including scrutiny of the case notes and drug chart, thorough physical examination and interpretation of appropriate investigations, including laboratory tests and imaging (Figure 2.6).

Is this acute or chronic kidney disease?

In this respect, much useful information may be gleaned from the patient notes, from previous biochemistry reports and from GP records, which may save a great deal of unnecessary investigation. Clues from the history and examination include evidence of long-standing diabetes and/or hypertension, though uraemic symptoms in themselves may be modest and/or non-specific. Anaemia, hypocalcaemia and hyperphosphataemia are typical of CKD but not universal. The most useful clue comes from previous creatinine measurements, if these can be found. Reduced renal size and cortical thickness on ultrasound is a feature of CKD, although renal size is generally preserved in patients with diabetes.

Has obstruction been excluded?

Careful urological evaluation is mandatory if the cause of AKI is not otherwise apparent, and this includes enquiry about previous stones or symptoms of bladder outflow obstruction and palpation for a palpable bladder. Anuria is an important clue, as this is otherwise unusual in AKI. Renal ultrasound is the method of choice to detect dilatation of the renal pelvis and calyces, although obstruction may be present without dilatation, particularly in cases of malignancy.

Is the patient euvolaemic?

Intravascular volume depletion is indicated by low venous pressure and a postural fall in BP, whereas volume overload manifests as raised venous pressure and pulmonary crepitations. Circumstances leading to pre-renal AKI are almost invariably associated with high levels of plasma antidiuretic hormone, leading to increased tubular reabsorption of both water and urea and a disproportional increase in the plasma urea:creatinine ratio. However, plasma urea may also be raised in the setting of increased catabolism due, for example, to sepsis or corticosteroid therapy, or protein load due, for example, to upper gastrointestinal (GI) bleeding. Typically, in pre-renal AKI there is avid retention of sodium and water, leading to low urinary sodium concentration. In clinical practice, however, the

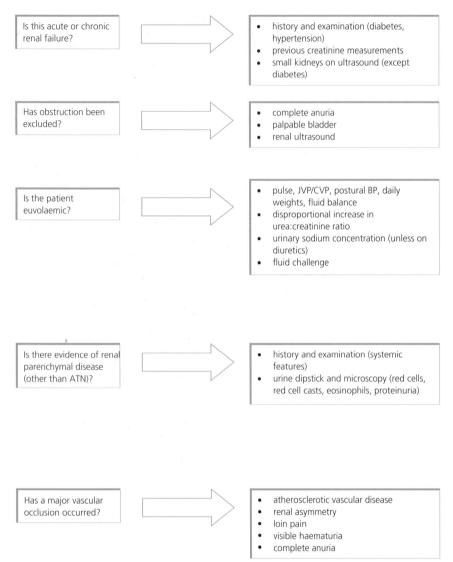

Is this acute or chronic renal failure?	• history and examination (diabetes, hypertension) • previous creatinine measurements • small kidneys on ultrasound (except diabetes)
Has obstruction been excluded?	• complete anuria • palpable bladder • renal ultrasound
Is the patient euvolaemic?	• pulse, JVP/CVP, postural BP, daily weights, fluid balance • disproportional increase in urea:creatinine ratio • urinary sodium concentration (unless on diuretics) • fluid challenge
Is there evidence of renal parenchymal disease (other than ATN)?	• history and examination (systemic features) • urine dipstick and microscopy (red cells, red cell casts, eosinophils, proteinuria)
Has a major vascular occlusion occurred?	• atherosclerotic vascular disease • renal asymmetry • loin pain • visible haematuria • complete anuria

Figure 2.6 Differential diagnosis. JVP: Jugular venous pressure; CVP: central venous pressure; BP: blood pressure; ATN: acute tubular necrosis.

use of diuretics frequently renders urinary indices uninterpretable. If doubt remains, a fluid challenge should be undertaken, but under continuous medical observation (jugular venous pressure, BP, urine volume) as life-threatening pulmonary oedema may be induced, particularly if the patient is oliguric or anuric (Figure 2.7).

Is there evidence of renal parenchymal disease (other than ATN)?

Intrinsic renal disease other than ATN is uncommon, but must always be excluded as this has important management implications. The history and examination may suggest an underlying multisystem disease, and it is helpful to ask specifically about rashes, arthralgia or myalgia. A careful drug history enquiring specifically about use of antibiotics and NSAIDs (widely available without prescription) is essential, as these commonly used drugs can cause acute interstitial nephritis. Urine dipstick and microscopy are mandatory to avoid missing a renal inflammatory process. Urinary catheterization can cause haematuria, and the concentrated

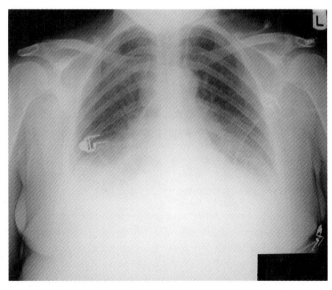

Figure 2.7 Chest X-ray showing pulmonary oedema.

urine seen in AKI can be rich in casts. The presence of significant blood or protein on dipstick (3+/4+), or dysmorphic red cells, red cell casts (suggestive of glomerulonephritis) or eosinophils (suggestive of acute interstitial nephritis) on microscopy – assuming that competent urinary microscopy is available – warrants prompt referral to a nephrologist.

Has a major vascular occlusion occurred?

AKI is common in older patients, as is coexistent atherosclerotic vascular disease, which frequently involves the renal arteries. Whereas occlusion of a normal renal artery results in loin pain and haematuria, occlusion of a previously stenosed renal artery may be clinically silent, leaving the patient dependent upon a single functioning kidney. An important clue is renal asymmetry on imaging, particularly in a patient with vascular disease elsewhere. In this setting, AKI may be precipitated by occlusion (thrombotic or embolic) of the artery supplying the remaining kidney. Risk factors include use of ACE inhibitors and diuretics in the context of renal artery stenosis, hypotension (either drug-induced or due to volume depletion) or instrumentation of the renal artery or aorta. The diagnosis is supported by the presence of complete anuria. Occlusion of a previously normal renal artery is relatively rare, most commonly arising as a consequence of embolization from a central source.

Investigations

A scheme of investigation is shown in Table 2.5, though clearly this should be tailored to individual circumstances. It is unnecessary, for example, to request a full battery of immunological tests in a patient with post-operative ATN or urinary tract obstruction, but this is appropriate if the diagnosis is uncertain or a renal inflammatory condition is suspected (e.g. in the setting of proteinuria and/or haematuria).

Management principles

Management of established AKI encompasses general measures irrespective of cause (Box 2.1) and specific therapies targeted to the particular aetiology, the latter being beyond the scope of this

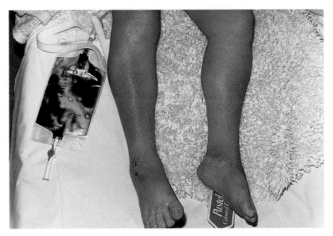

Figure 2.8 Acute kidney injury due to rhabdomyolysis (chocolate-coloured urine can be seen in the catheter bag).

Table 2.5 Scheme of investigation.

	Test	Comments
Urinalysis	Dipstick for blood and/or protein	Suggestive of a renal inflammatory process
	Microscopy for cells, casts, crystals	Red cell casts diagnostic in glomerulonephritis
Biochemistry	Serial urea, creatinine, electrolytes	Important metabolic consequences of acute kidney injury include hyperkalaemia, metabolic acidosis, hypocalcaemia, hyperphosphataemia
	Blood gas analysis, serum bicarbonate	
	Creatine kinase, myoglobinuria	Markedly elevated creatine kinase and myoglobinuria suggestive of rhabdomyolysis (Figure 2.8)
	C-reactive protein	Non-specific marker of infection or inflammation
	Serum immunoglobulins, serum protein electrophoresis, Bence Jones proteinuria	Immune paresis, monoclonal band on serum protein electrophoresis and Bence Jones proteinuria suggestive of myeloma
Haematology	Full blood count, blood film	Eosinophilia may be present in acute interstitial nephritis, cholesterol embolization or vasculitis
		Thrombocytopenia and red cell fragments suggestive of thrombotic microangiopathy
	Coagulation studies	Disseminated intravascular coagulation associated with sepsis
Immunology	ANA	ANA positive in SLE and other autoimmune disorders; anti-dsDNA antibodies more specific for SLE
	Anti-dsDNA antibody	
	ANCA	Associated with systemic vasculitis c-ANCA and anti-PR3 antibodies associated with Wegener's granulomatosis; p-ANCA and anti-MPO antibodies present in microscopic polyangiitis
	PR3 antibodies	
	MPO antibodies	
	Complement levels	Low in SLE, acute post-infectious glomerulonephritis, essential cryoglobulinaemia
	Antiglomerular basement membrane antibodies	Present in Goodpasture's disease
	Antistreptolysin O and anti-DNase B titres	Elevated following streptococcal infection
Virology	Hepatitis B and C; HIV	Important implications for infection control within the dialysis area
Radiology	Renal ultrasound	Gives important information about renal size, symmetry, evidence of obstruction

SLE, systemic lupus erythematosus; ANA, anti-nuclear antibody; anti-dsDNA antibody: anti-double-stranded DNA antibodies; ANCA, antineutrophil cytoplasmic antibody; PR3, antiproteinase 3; MPO, antimyeloperoxidase.

Table 2.6 Treatment of acute kidney injury.

Treatment	Evidence of benefit	Comment
Loop diuretics	No difference in renal recovery or mortality compared with placebo	May promote diuresis in oliguric AKI, but may be ototoxic in high doses
Dopamine	No difference in mortality or need for dialysis compared with placebo	Potential adverse effects include tachycardia, extravasation necrosis and peripheral gangrene
Natriuretic peptides	No difference in dialysis-free survival compared with placebo	
Renal replacement therapy	No significant difference in dialysis-dependency or mortality between continuous and intermittent renal replacement therapy	Continuous renal replacement therapy is less likely to provoke haemodynamic instability

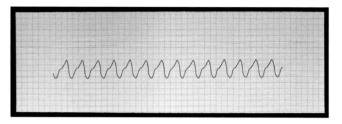

Figure 2.9 An ECG showing sinusoidal waves, in an acute kidney injury patient with a plasma potassium of 7.9 mmol/L.

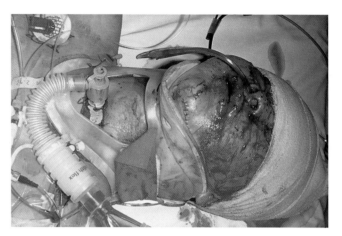

Figure 2.10 A trauma victim: Massive exsanguination can lead to acute kidney injury.

chapter. No pharmacological therapy has been shown to limit the progression of or speed up the recovery from AKI; indeed, some drugs may be harmful (Table 2.6).

Box 2.1 **Box Management principles in acute kidney injury**

- Identify and correct pre-renal and post-renal factors
- Optimize cardiac output and renal blood flow
- Review medication: cease nephrotoxic agents; adjust doses where appropriate; monitor levels where appropriate
- Accurately monitor fluid intake and output and daily bodyweight
- Identify and treat acute complications (hyperkalaemia, acidosis, hyperphosphataemia, pulmonary oedema)
- Optimize nutritional support: adequate calories but minimize nitrogenous waste production; potassium restriction (Figure 2.9)
- Identify and aggressively treat infection; minimize indwelling lines; remove bladder catheter if anuric
- Identify and treat bleeding tendency (Figure 2.10): prophylaxis with proton pump inhibitor or H_2-antagonist; transfuse if required; avoid aspirin
- Initiate dialysis before uraemic complications emerge

Summary

AKI is common and carries a high mortality rate. It is crucial to identify at-risk patients and institute appropriate preventative measures. Management of AKI includes prevention of life-threatening metabolic consequences and early referral to a nephrologist where appropriate (Box 2.1).

Further reading

Allen A (2002) The aetiology of acute renal failure. In: Glynne P, Allen A, Pusey CD (eds), *Acute Renal Failure in Practice*, pp. 39–45. Imperial College Press, London.

Firth JD (2005) The clinical approach to the patient with acute renal failure. In: Davison AM, Cameron JS, Grunfeld J-P *et al.* (eds), *Oxford Textbook of Clinical Nephrology*, 3rd edn, pp. 1465–93. Oxford University Press, Oxford.

Kellum JA (2012) Treating acute renal failure: A guide to the evidence, http://www.bmjlearning.com.

Kidney Disease: Improving Global Outcomes (KDIGO) Acute Kidney Injury Work Group. KDIGO Clinical Practice Guideline for Acute Kidney Injury. *Kidney Int.*, Suppl. 2012; **2**: 1–138.

Lameire N, Van Biesen W, Vanholder R (2005) Acute renal failure. *Lancet* **365**: 417–430.

CHAPTER 3

Prevalence, Detection, Evaluation and Management of Chronic Kidney Disease

Penny Ackland

Nunhead Surgery, Nunhead Grove, South East London, UK

OVERVIEW

- It is important to be able to identify those with early **chronic kidney disease (CKD)**, firstly because CKD has a very strong association with the risk of death, cardiovascular disease and hospitalization, and secondly, in order to attempt to prevent/delay the progression to end-stage renal disease (ESRD).

- In relation to the management of CKD, important factors to consider are the rate of change of kidney function and whether there is proteinuria or haematuria. The presence of other comorbidities, current or recent drug history, family history and the age of the patient are additional factors that need to be taken into account.

- If estimated glomerular filtration rate (eGFR) is $<60\,mL/min/1.73\,m^2$ in the first test, retest within two weeks to exclude causes of acute deterioration of glomerular filtration rate (GFR).

- Significant progression of CKD is defined as a decline in eGFR of $>5\,mL/min/1.73\,m^2$ within 1 year, or $>10\,mL/min/1.73\,m^2$ within five years.

- All CKD patients should be checked for proteinuria.

- In people without diabetes, albuminuria/proteinuria is considered clinically significant when the albumin:creatinine ratio (ACR) is $\geqq 30\,mg/mmol$.

- In people with diabetes, consider microalbuminuria of an $ACR > 2.5\,mg/mmol$ in men and $>3.5\,mg/mmol$ in women to be clinically significant.

- A nephrological referral should be considered (a) if there is significant proteinuria ($ACR \geqq 70$, or protein:creatinine ratio ($PCR) \geqq 100$) with or without haematuria or (b) if the $ACR \geqq 30$ or $PCR \geqq 50$ with haematuria.

- If a young adult has haematuria (cola-coloured!) and an intercurrent illness (usually an upper respiratory tract infection), they should be suspected of having acute glomerulonephritis.

- In general, people in stages 4 and 5 CKD, with or without diabetes, should be considered for specialist assessment. However, at an earlier stage, other factors – including proteinuria, haematuria, poorly controlled hypertension, rate of change of eGFR and consideration as to whether the rate of progression of eGFR would make renal replacement therapy likely within the person's lifetime – would all influence the need for referral.

Introduction

Until recently, the care of kidney patients has been largely under the domain of nephrologists in secondary care. However, the increasing number of people diagnosed with chronic kidney disease (CKD), previously termed chronic renal failure, along with the more active treatment of end-stage renal disease (many more people have access to dialysis now than even a decade or so ago) means that not only has more of the care been streamlined into nurse-led clinics, but the earlier stages of renal disease are now being managed in the community by GPs.

This latter strategy means that an ever-wider group of healthcare professionals is obliged to have an understanding and basic knowledge of issues in relation to patients with CKD. The aim of this chapter is to discuss the prevalence, detection, evaluation and management of this condition.

Prevalence and staging of chronic kidney disease

Several epidemiologic studies have indicated that there is a high prevalence of CKD in the general population. The survey conducted by the Centers for Disease Control and Prevention in the United States from 1999 to 2004 suggested that up to 16.8% of the adult population have CKD (Centers for Disease Control and Prevention 2007). Another US study, the National Health and Nutrition Survey (NHANES III), based on data from 15 635 adults and including measurements of creatinine, urine albumin:creatinine ratio (ACR) and estimate glomerular filtration rate (eGFR), estimated that the prevalence of CKD was 11% (equating in 2003 to 19.2 million adults in the United States) (Coresh *et al.* 2003; Figure 3.1). Data from the United Kingdom suggests a similarly high prevalence of CKD in the general adult population (Anandarajah *et al.* 2005).

Despite the high prevalence, only a minority of those with CKD will progress to end-stage renal disease (ESRD) (Hallen *et al.* 2006) and the majority of CKD patients will be identified and managed within the primary care setting. It is important to be able to identify those with early CKD, firstly because CKD has a very strong association with the risk of death, cardiovascular disease and hospitalization (Figure 3.2; Table 3.1), and secondly in order to attempt to prevent/delay the progression to ESRD, which is associated with considerable morbidity and a high mortality (UK Renal Registry 2009), as well as affecting quality of life. Furthermore, costs of

ABC of Kidney Disease, Second edition.
Edited by David Goldsmith, Satish Jayawardene and Penny Ackland.
© 2013 John Wiley & Sons, Ltd. Published 2013 by John Wiley & Sons, Ltd.

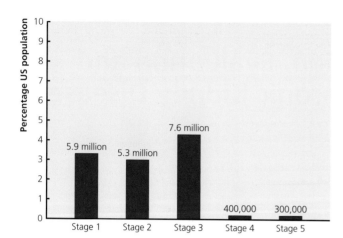

Figure 3.1 NHANES III data showing the prevalence of CKD Stages 1 to 5 in the United States in 2003. (*Source:* Coresh *et al.* 2003.)

ESRD are considerable. In the United Kingdom, the absolute cost per patient is around £30,000–£35,000 per year for haemodialysis patients, and around £20,000–£25,000 per year for peritoneal dialysis patients.

In order to help in the early identification of patients, and enable stratification of risk and management, CKD has been categorized into stages dependent on the eGFR, whether other evidence of kidney damage is present and whether or not there is proteinuria.

In September 2008, the NICE guideline on CKD (NICE 2008) updated the staging of CKD. The previous stage 3 (30–59 ml/min) was subdivided into stage 3A with an eGFR of between 45 and 59 ml/min/1.73 m^2, and stage 3B with an eGFR of between 30 and 44 mL/min/1.73 m^2. In addition, it is recommended that the suffix 'p' be placed after the stage to denote the presence of proteinuria, where proteinuria is defined as urinary ACR $\geq$ 30 mg/mmol or PCR $\geq$ 50 mg/mmol. The rationale for these changes was an increasing realization that most of the complications associated with CKD showed a rapid increase in prevalence in patients with an eGFR of <45 ml/min, and that the prognosis for patients with proteinuria was very much worse compared to those without proteinuria (Table 3.2).

Table 3.1 Independent predictive variables for combined endpoints of CV death, myocardial infarction and stroke. (Source: Reprinted from The Lancet, HOPE Study Investigators, 2000; 355: 253–259, with permission from Elsevier.)

Variable	Hazard Ratio
Microalbuminuria	1.59
Creatinine > 123.76 mmol/L	1.40
CAD	1.51
PVD	1.49
Diabetes mellitus	1.42
Male	1.20
Age	1.03
Waist:Hip ratio	1.13

CAD, Coronary Artery Disease; PVD, Peripheral Vascular Disease.

Table 3.2 Stages of chronic kidney disease and frequency of estimated glomerular filtration rate testing (NICE 2008).

Stage	eGFR (ml/min/1.73 m^2)	Description	Typical testing frequency[a]
1	$\geq$ 90	Normal or increased GFR, with other evidence of kidney damage	12 monthly
2	60–89	Slight decrease in GFR, with other evidence of kidney damage	
3A	45–59	Moderate decrease in GFR, with or without other evidence of kidney damage	6 monthly
3B	30–44		
4	15–29	Severe decrease in GFR, with or without other evidence of kidney damage	3 monthly
5	< 15	End stage renal failure	6 weekly

Test eGFR
- Annually in all at risk groups.
- During intercurrent illness and perioperatively in all patients with CKD.
- The exact frequency should depend on the clinical situation. The frequency of testing may be reduced where eGFR levels remain very stable but will need to be increased if there is rapid progression.

GFR, glomerular filtration rate; eGFR, estimated glomerular filtration rate; CKD, chronic kidney disease; ESRF, end stage renal failure.

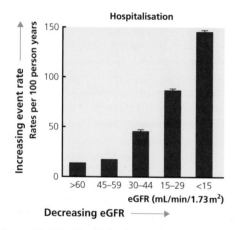

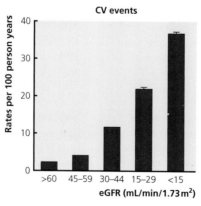

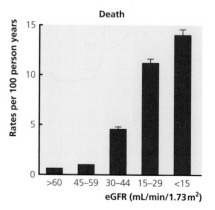

Figure 3.2 Risk of hospitalization, cardiovascular events and death with respect to renal function (eGFR). (*Source:* Go *et al.* 2004.)

Detection

CKD is often asymptomatic in its early stages. Kidney disease may be detected (whether routinely or as part of an investigative procedure) by:

- blood tests for creatinine/eGFR – routine or investigative;
- urine tests for albuminuria/proteinuria/haematuria – may be routine (change of GP, insurance medical, etc.) but also investigative. All hypertensive patients should have urinary ACR checks and urinalysis for haematuria (NICE 2011), while all diabetics should have first-pass urine tests for ACR (NICE 2009);
- family history – for those who have relatives with polycystic kidney disease or other rarer causes of hereditary renal disease (such as Alport's syndrome);
- renal imaging – in general, renal disease could be picked up by screening for other problems, e.g. coincidentally during ultrasonography for suspected gallstones. Ultrasound may also detect reflux nephropathy in babies in utero, or in the neonate.

In view of the high prevalence of CKD, it is becoming increasingly necessary to find a means to develop a 'renal risk score' in order to help identify those at risk of progressive CKD, as well as those who would benefit from referral to a nephrologist. Unfortunately, although such scores have indeed been devised (Halbesma *et al.* 2011), none is robust enough to be adopted into routine clinical management (Taal 2011). This is partly because there are a large number of CKD risk factors/markers (Table 3.3), which will affect the sensitivity of a simple, universally applicable scoring system. Over 75% of CKD patients will have either diabetes, hypertension or are aged over 65 years. Data from NHANES III showed about 25% of CKD cases had diabetes, 75% had hypertension, while 11% of all patients over 65 years who did not have diabetes or hypertension had CKD (Figure 3.3). It follows that an increasing prevalence of these factors parallels a proportionate rise in CKD prevalence.

According to NICE clinical guideline 73 (NICE 2008), people should be offered testing for CKD if they have any of the following risk factors:

- diabetes
- hypertension
- cardiovascular disease (ischaemic heart disease, chronic heart failure, peripheral vascular disease or cerebrovascular disease)
- structural renal tract disease, renal calculi or prostatic hypertrophy
- multisystem diseases with potential kidney involvement, e.g. systemic lupus erythematosus (SLE)
- family history of stage 5 CKD or hereditary kidney disease
- opportunistic detection of haematuria or proteinuria.

Evaluation

For the majority of patients with CKD there is no, or very slow, progression of renal impairment, and only a small percentage reach end-stage renal disease. In relation to the management of CKD, it is first necessary to take a good history, which will include concurrent or recent drug history as well as family history (e.g.

Table 3.3 Risk markers/factors for chronic kidney disease.

Non-modifiable	Modifiable
Old age (S)	Systemic hypertension (I, P)
Male sex (S)	Diabetes mellitus (I, P)
Race/ethnicity (S)	Proteinuria (P)
Genetic predisposition (S)	Dyslipidaemia (I, P)
Family history (S)	Smoking (I, P)
Low birth weight (S)	Obesity (I, P)
	Alcohol consumption (I, P)
	Low socio-economic status (S)
	Infections/Infestations (I)
	Drugs and herbs/analgesic abuse (I)
	Autoimmune diseases/obstructive uropathy/ stones (I)

S, Susceptibility factor, I, Initiation factor, P, Progression factor.

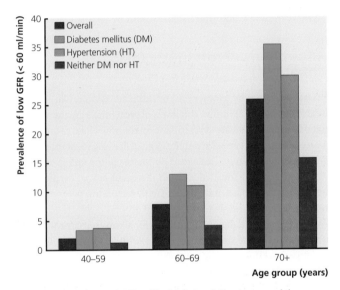

Figure 3.3 Prevalence of GFR < 60 mL/min in relation to age and the presence or absence of DM or HT. (*Source:* Coresh *et al.* 2003.)

for polycystic kidney disease and Alport's syndrome). Important factors to evaluate also include the rate of change of kidney function and whether there is proteinuria or haematuria. The presence of other comorbidities (such as diabetes, hypertension, SLE) and the age of the patient are additional factors that need to be considered. Even though a decline in GFR with age is normal, there is currently no consensus around which level of GFR is considered 'normal' at a certain age. The eGFR takes age into consideration, but does not fully correct for the natural ageing process.

Creatinine/Estimated glomerular filtration rate

- When checking eGFR, bear in mind ethnicity, weight, age, muscle mass, gender, diet (protein meal) and exercise.
- NICE clinical guideline 73 (NICE 2008) advises the use of the simplified MDRD equation to estimate eGFR. Since eGFR may be less reliable in certain situations (such as acute kidney injury, pregnancy, oedematous states, muscle wasting disorders, amputees

and malnutrition), the serum creatinine should be considered as well as the eGFR.

- With Afro-Caribbean or African ethnicity, the eGFR should be corrected by multiplying by 1.21. Validation of the eGFR has not been well established for those of Asian or Chinese ethnicity.
- Caution in eGFR interpretation should be used for people with extremes of muscle mass, for those who have taken creatine supplements, or if the patient performed heavy exercise before their blood test.
- Protein meals or supplements may also affect the eGFR, and meat should be avoided for at least 12 hours before an eGFR blood test.
- If eGFR is <60 ml/min/1.73 m^2 in the first test, retest within two weeks to exclude causes of acute deterioration of GFR.
- To identify progressive CKD, obtain a minimum of three eGFR estimations over a period of not less than 90 days. Progressive CKD is defined as a decline in eGFR of >5 ml/min/1.73 m^2 within one year, or >10 ml/min/1.73 m^2 within five years.

Albuminuria/Proteinuria (also see Chapter 1)

Proteinuria can be glomerular or tubular. Glomerular protein largely consists of albumin, and levels of proteinuria greater than 1 g per day usually indicate glomerular proteinuria, which results from a breakdown in the integrity of the glomerular basement membrane and, more specifically, damage to podocytes in the membrane.

Proteinuria is associated with an increased risk of cardiovascular disease and is an independent risk factor for progression of renal disease.

All CKD patients should be checked for albuminuria/proteinuria. This may easily be detected by testing urine using reagent strips, but these are not usually as sensitive as sending the sample to the biochemistry lab for measurement of ACR (albumin:creatinine ratio) or PCR (protein:creatinine ratio). The ACR has greater sensitivity than PCR for low levels of proteinuria and is usually the preferred test, but nephrologists still tend to use PCR more than ACR. The opposite is true among diabetologists, who more commonly use ACR so that they can detect the very earliest stages of diabetic nephropathy, which may be amenable to treatment (Table 3.4).

- If the initial ACR is ≥ 30 mg/mmol and <70 mg/mmol, a further early-morning sample for ACR should be sent for confirmation. If the initial sample is >70 mg/mmol, no repeat sample is necessary.
- In people without diabetes, proteinuria is considered clinically significant when the ACR is ≥ 30 mg/mmol.
- However, in people with diabetes, consider microalbuminuria with an ACR > 2.5 mg/mmol in men and >3.5 mg/mmol in women to be clinically significant.

Table 3.4 Approximate equivalent values of ACR, PCR, and urinary protein excretion. (*Source:* NICE 2008.).

ACR (mg/mmol)	PCR (mg/mmol)	Urinary protein excretion g/24 hr
30	50	0.5
70	100	1

Haematuria (also see Chapter 1)

Haematuria can either be glomerular (from the kidney) or extra-glomerular (from a urological source).

- When testing for haematuria, urinary reagent strips should be used rather than urine microscopy. This is partly because of the lack of availability of access to quality microscopic techniques with skilled operators and partly because of the need for the microscopy testing to be performed on a relatively fresh sample of urine. Dipstick urinalysis has the advantages of simplicity and accessibility.
- Microscopic haematuria is now more aptly termed non-visible haematuria (NVH). This can be subdivided into symptomatic NVH with the presence of lower urinary tract symptoms, or asymptomatic NVH.
- If there is a positive urinary reagent strip test of 1+ or more of blood, confirmation with a reagent strip (as opposed to microscopically) should be made, and further evaluation will be necessary. Trace haematuria should be considered negative.
- Any episode of visible haematuria or symptomatic NVH in the absence of a urinary tract infection (UTI) or transient cause is considered significant. Persistence of asymptomatic NVH (defined as at least two out of three positive NVH dipsticks) is also considered significant.
- Investigate symptomatic and persistent asymptomatic haematuria by (i) excluding UTIs or other transient causes; (ii) checking creatinine/eGFR; (iii) sending urine for ACR or PCR on a random sample [an approximation to the 24-hour urine albumin or protein excretion (in mg) can be obtained by multiplying the ratio (in mg/mmol) $\times$ 10]; (iv) measuring blood pressure (BP) (BAUS/RA 2008).
- All patients with significant visible or symptomatic non-visible haematuria, and patients over the age of 40 years with asymptomatic non-visible haematuria, should be considered for **urological referral**. An exception of referring directly to a nephrologist may be a young adult who has haematuria (cola-coloured!) and an intercurrent illness (usually an upper respiratory tract infection), and who is suspected of having acute glomerulonephritis.
- A **nephrological referral** should be considered (a) if there is significant proteinuria (ACR ≥ 70, or PCR ≥ 100) with or without haematuria, or (b) if the ACR ≥ 30 or PCR ≥ 50 with haematuria.
- For those with haematuria but no proteinuria, there should be annual testing for haematuria, albuminuria/proteinuria, eGFR and BP monitoring, as long as the haematuria persists. An adult under the age of 40 years with hypertension and isolated haematuria (i.e. in the absence of proteinuria) should be referred to a nephrologist. The two most common causes of this scenario are hypertensive nephropathy and IgA nephropathy.

Non-visible haematuria is seen in 3–6% of the normal population. A recent 22-year retrospective study of over 1.2 million young adults found a substantially increased risk for treated ESRD attributed to primary glomerular disease in individuals with persistent asymptomatic isolated non-visible haematuria compared to those without. However, the incidence and absolute risk of ESRD remains quite low (Vivante *et al.* 2011).

Renal imaging (also see Chapter 1)

Renal ultrasound should be offered to all people with CKD who (i) have progressive CKD, (ii) have visible or persistent non-visible haematuria, (iii) have symptoms of urinary tract obstruction, (iv) have a family history of polycystic kidney disease and are over 20 years old, (v) have stage 4 or 5 CKD and (vi) require a kidney biopsy.

More specialist/other renal screening tests for underlying cause of chronic kidney disease

- There are several complementary different ways to screen for the presence of renovascular disease (which is typically atheroscleroticin most adults) – including **MR scanning, CT scanning and Doppler US screening**. Check with your local radiology department to see which is favoured for screening. See Chapter 8 for more detailed information.
- **Serum immunoglobulins/protein electrophoresis/serum-free light chains** may be requested to screen for myeloma.
- **Auto-antibodies: ANA, dsDNA, ANCA, anti-GBM antibody.** ANA and dsDNA are useful screening tools for SLE and may indicate underlying lupus nephritis as the cause of CKD. Screening for possible vasculitis should include a request for antinuclear cytoplasmic antibody (ANCA). Likewise, a positive anti-GBM antibody may indicate underlying Goodpasture's disease.
- **Complement levels** both C3 and C4 levels are often reduced in active SLE, and low C3 levels may indicate underlying mesangio-capillary glomerulonephritis (MCGN).
- **Virology** several glomerulonephritides may be driven by viruses and other infectious agents (e.g. Hep B, Hep C, HIV). A positive

HIV test may suggest underlying HIV-associated nephropathy (HIVAN), which presents with proteinuria +/− renal impairment and almost exclusively occurs in black people.

- **Renal biopsy** In patients with renal impairment and/or proteinuria of more than 1 g per day (PCR > 100), a renal biopsy may be required to elucidate the cause of underlying CKD, provided this is technically feasible. (Relative contraindications may be extreme obesity, small kidneys of less than 9 cm, etc.)
- **Genetic testing** Although two gene mutations (PKD1 and PKD2) have been identified in patients with polycystic kidney disease, the test is not widely available, and its utility remains questionable. There are potentially some instances when this test may be useful (e.g. in a family when the mutation is already known), but widespread adoption of this test is not considered appropriate at the present time.

Management

The management of CKD varies according to the stage of CKD (Figure 3.4) and can be divided into both general and specific measures.

General

(i) **Blood pressure control**

BP control is mandatory in any patient with CKD, firstly to slow down the progress of renal impairment, and secondly, to reduce the risk of cardiovascular events. The beneficial effects that BP control has on the kidney are largely mediated via a reduction in intraglomerular capillary pressure to preserve the integrity of the glomerulus. In general, the aim

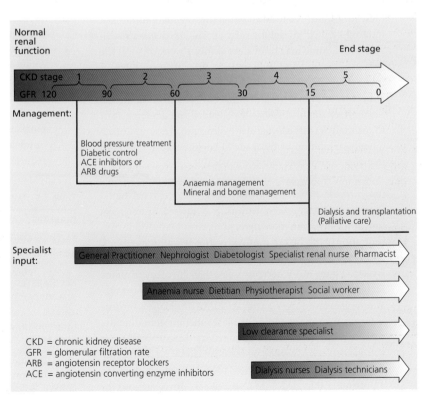

Figure 3.4 The lifecycle of the CKD patient. *Source:* Ackland P (2009) *Journal of Renal Nursing* **1**(1): 26–7 with permission from MA Healthcare.

should be to keep the BP below 140/90; however, in people with diabetes and CKD, or when the ACR $\geq$ 70 mg/mmol, one should aim for a BP below 130/80. However, the evidence that this more stringent target is truly beneficial is weak, so care must be taken especially in vulnerable groups such as the elderly. NICE now recommends that a diagnosis of hypertension be made using 24-hour ambulatory blood pressure monitoring (ABPM), which should be offered to patients if the clinic BP is 140/90 mmHg or higher (NICE 2011).

(ii) **Diabetes control**

Data from the ADVANCE trial have shown fairly convincingly that good glycaemic control can slow down the progression of renal disease (ADVANCE Collaborative Group et al. 2008). This was also confirmed in the UK PD study. However over-aggressive management of diabetes leading to increased hypoglycaemic episodes is harmful so this should be carefully avoided.

(iii) **Angiotensin converting enzyme inhibition (ACEI)/ Angiotensin receptor blockade (ARB)**

ACEIs and ARBs exert a number of positive benefits in patients with CKD. Specifically, they lower BP, they reduce proteinuria and they preserve renal function in the longer term. Therefore, part of their action is mediated via a reduction in BP and intraglomerular pressure, but it is now apparent that other mechanisms play a part in their renoprotective effects. Their selective action on the efferent arteriole may reduce intraglomerular pressure over and above the reduction in systemic arterial pressure. In addition to its vasoconstrictive action, angiotensin II may induce other pathogenetic mechanisms, such as mesangial hypertrophy. Thus, reducing the levels, or blocking angiotensin II, may explain why ACEIs or ARBs are renoprotective. Following the introduction of these drugs, there may be an initial small reduction in eGFR induced by their intraglomerular effects, and a small rise in serum creatinine may be evident within a week or so. If the increase in creatinine level exceeds 30%, the possibility of underlying renovascular disease should be entertained. This is because a kidney that is ischaemic due to a significant renal artery stenosis is heavily dependent on angiotensin II to maintain its intraglomerular hydrostatic pressure. Consequently, inhibition or blockade of angiotensin II will result in a disproportionate reduction in eGFR.

With the risk of exacerbating renal failure with ACEI/ARB use in those patients who may have reduced renal blood flow due to renal artery stenosis, it is advised to test renal function (including measurement of serum potassium concentration) both before starting treatment with these drugs, and 1–2 weeks after any dose increase. No dose modification is needed if the eGFR decrease is less than 25% (or creatinine increase is <30%). If the eGFR decreases by $\geq$ 25% (or creatinine increase $\geq$ 30%) after ACEI/ARB initiation or dose increase, then other causes of renal function deterioration, such as nonsteroidal anti-inflammatory drugs (NSAIDs) or volume depletion, need to be excluded, and if no other cause is found, the ACEI/ARB will need to be stopped or reduced to a previously tolerated dose (NICE 2008). Investigations for

peripheral vascular disease and renal artery dopplers looking for stenosis may be considered.

There is strong evidence that:

- proteinuria can be reduced (and even reversed), and the progression of CKD can be slowed, by the use of ACEIs or ARBs in diabetic nephropathy (Lewis et al. 1993);
- the risk of CKD progression can also be reduced amongst non-diabetic CKD patients with proteinuria of > 1g per day (or PCR of >100 mg/mmol) by treating with ACEIs or ARBs (Ruggenenti et al. 1998).

The latest suggestions from the Global Guidelines body Kidney Disease Improving Global Outcomes (KDIGO) now suggest that wherever micro'albuminuria is detected, whether in diabetic or non'diabetic patients, the use of ACE inhibitors, and ARBs, should be considered (Table 3.5).

When using ACEIs/ARBs, it is important to monitor renal function and potassium levels, and titrate the drugs to the maximum tolerated therapeutic dose before adding a second-line agent. ACEIs/ARBs should not be started if the serum potassium is significantly above the normal reference range, and other factors that promote hyperkalaemia need to be excluded and treated. More frequent monitoring of serum potassium is required if medication that promotes hyperkalaemia is being taken, and the ACEIs/ARBs should be discontinued if the serum potassium rises to $\geq$ 6 mmol/l.

Lowering dietary salt intake reduces BP and lowers proteinuria more effectively than an ACEI, and augments the action of the ACEI if its restriction is used in conjunction with it. It is more effective, in general, in the black population.

(iv) **Correct dehydration**

(v) **Drugs**

eGFR will need monitoring in patients prescribed known nephrotoxic drugs such as lithium and calcineurin inhibitors (ciclosporin and tacrolimus). Those receiving long-term NSAIDs should have at least annual checks on renal function. An uncommon allergic response to protein pump inhibitors and some antibiotics can lead to acute or chronic interstitial nephritis, which is usually reversible on stopping the offending drug. Since many drugs are excreted via the kidneys, renal failure may lead to increased blood concentrations of a number of medications, including opiates and digoxin, and reduced doses are often required.

Table 3.5 Use of ACEI/ARBs in people with CKD. (Source: NICE 2008).

DIABETES

ACR > 2.5 mg/mmol (men) or > 3.5 mg/mmol (women) with or without hypertension	Offer ACEI or ARB

NO DIABETES

Hypertension and ACR < 30 mg/mmol	Offer choice of antihypertensive treatment according to NICE (2006)
Hypertension and ACR > 30 mg/mmol	Offer ACEI or ARB
ACR $\geq$ 70 mg/mmol	Offer ACEI or ARB

ACR, albumin:creatinine ratio; ACEI, angiotensin converting enzyme inhibitor; ARB, angiotensin receptor blocker.

(vi) **Manage cardiovascular health**

Statins should be used for the primary prevention of cardiovascular disease in the same way as in people without CKD. In the SHARP study, patients with CKD were randomized to lipid lowering therapy (simvastatin or simvastatin/ezetimibe) versus placebo. The primary outcome (major atherosclerotic events defined as a composite of coronary death, myocardial infarction, non-haemorrhagic stroke or any revascularization) was reduced by 17% (Baigent *et al.* 2011).

Both statins (irrespective of baseline lipid values) and antiplatelet drugs should also be used for the secondary prevention of cardiovascular disease. However, the prescriber should be aware that there is an increased risk of minor bleeding in people with CKD given multiple antiplatelet drugs.

Patients with CKD should be advised on the need for regular exercise, maintaining a healthy weight and stopping smoking.

(vii) **Malnutrition**

Several animal studies have indicated a slower progression of renal impairment with very low protein diets. Unfortunately the protein restriction required to protect renal function was found to be impractical for patients: it has the risk of exacerbating malnutrition. Nowadays, a normal, but not excessive, protein intake of 1 g/kg/day is recommended.

Dietary advice on protein, potassium and phosphate intake may be needed for some people with progressive CKD.

(viii) **Anaemia**

See Chapter 5.

(ix) **CKD-Mineral and Bone Disorder (CKD-MBD)**

See Chapter 4.

(x) **Acidosis and hyperkalaemia**

See Chapter 4.

(xi) **Manage fluid overload**

Manage fluid overload while avoiding deterioration in renal function from diuretic use. See Chapter 4.

(xii) **Dialysis**

See Chapter 10.

(xiii) **Palliative care**

See Chapter 9.

Specific

(i) **Nephrotic syndrome** – steroids for minimal change nephropathy

(ii) **Crescentic glomerulonephritis/vasculitis** – steroids and cyclophosphamide

(iii) **Lupus nephritis** (depends on WHO class) – steroids and cyclophosphamide; mycophenolate

(iv) **HIVAN** – HAART therapy has been shown to help HIVAN

(v) **Myeloma** – chemotherapy (Dexamethasone/Thalidomide/Melphalan/Bortezomib), plus trials using high flux dialysis membranes, are in progress (EuLITE study)

(vi) **Drugs** – interstitial nephritis – stop offending medication, such as antibiotics, NSAIDs, proton pump inhibitors, and give steroids if still active.

Patients will need tailored education about their condition in order to help them understand and make informed choices about treatment. There will be a large group of patients, particularly in Stage 3A CKD, who will not experience significant deterioration in renal function but may suffer disproportionate anxiety about their health without adequate explanation.

Although the majority of CKD patients can be managed within the community, it is important to recognize those patients who would benefit from referral to a nephrologist. In certain cases discussing the management issues of a particular individual with a specialist may avoid the need for referral.

A patient's wishes and comorbidities need to be taken into account when referral is considered. In general, people in stages 4 and 5 CKD, with or without diabetes, should be considered for specialist assessment. However, at an earlier stage, other factors – including proteinuria, haematuria, poorly controlled hypertension, rate of change of eGFR and consideration as to whether the rate of progression of eGFR would make renal replacement therapy likely within the person's lifetime – would all influence the need for referral.

The NICE (2008) guideline on CKD suggests referral for the following groups of people with CKD:

- stages 4 and 5 CKD
- higher levels of proteinuria (ACR $\geq$ 70 mg/mmol) unless known to be due to diabetes and appropriately treated
- proteinuria (ACR $\geq$ 30 mg/mmol) together with haematuria
- rapidly declining eGFR (>5 ml/min/1.73 m^2 in one year, or >10 mL/min/1.73 m^2 within five years)
- hypertension that remains poorly controlled despite the use of at least four antihypertensive drugs at therapeutic doses
- people suspected of having rare or genetic causes of CKD
- suspected renal artery stenosis.

When under hospital care, a patient with CKD may attend either a general nephrology clinic, a low clearance clinic or undergo dialysis. Palliative treatment is an option for some patients with end-stage kidney failure, and management of these patients is often undertaken in the community alongside collaboration with renal/palliative care specialists.

References

ADVANCE Collaborative Group, Patel A, MacMahon S *et al.* (2008) Intensive blood glucose control and vascular outcomes in patients with type 2 diabetes. *N Engl J Med* **358**: 2560–2572.

Anandarajah S, Tai T, de Lusignan S *et al.* (2005) The validity of searching routinely collected general practice computer data to identify patients with chronic kidney disease (CKD): A manual review of 500 medical records. *Nephrol Dial Transplant* **20**: 2089–96.

Baigent C, Landray MJ, Reith C *et al.* (2011) SHARP Investigators: The effects of lowering LDL cholesterol with simvastatin plus ezetimibe in patients with chronic kidney disease (Study of Heart and Renal Protection): A randomised placebo-controlled trial. *Lancet* **377**: 2181–92.

BAUS/RA Guidelines (2008) *Joint Consensus Statement on the Initial Assessment of Haematuria* http://www.renal.org/Libraries/Other_Guidlines/Haematuria_-_RA-BAUS_consensus_guideline_2008.sflb.ashx.

Centers for Disease Control and Prevention (2007) Prevalence of chronic kidney disease and associated risk factors: United States, 1999–2004. *Morb Mortal Wkly Rep* **56**: 161–5.

Coresh J, Astor BC, Greene T, Eknoyan G, Levey AS (2003) Prevalence of chronic kidney disease and decreased kidney function in the adult US population: Third National Health and Nutrition Examination Survey. *Am J Kidney Dis* **41**: 1–12.

Go AS, Chertow GM, Fan D, McCulloch CE, Hsu CY (2004) Chronic kidney disease and the risks of death, cardiovascular events, and hospitalization. *N Engl J Med* **351**: 1296–305.

Halbesma N, Jansen DF, Heymans MW *et al.* (2011) PREVEND Study Group: Development and validation of a general population renal risk score. *Clin J Am Soc Nephrol* **6**: 1731–8.

Hallen SI, Dahl K, Oien CM *et al.* (2006) Follow-up of cross sectional health survey. *BMJ* **333**: 1047.

HOPE Study Investigators (2000) Effects of ramipril on cardiovascular and microvascular outcomes in people with diabetes mellitus: Results of the HOPE study and MICRO-HOPE substudy. *Lancet* **355**: 253–9. See Chapter 4.

Lewis EJ, Hunsicker LG, Bain RP, Rohde RD (1993) The effect of angiotensin-converting-enzyme inhibition on diabetic nephropathy. *N Engl J Med* **329**: 1456–62.

NICE (2006) Clinical Guideline 34: *Hypertension*, http://www.nice.org.uk/nicemedia/pdf/cg034quickrefguide.pdf.

NICE (2011) *Clinical Guideline 127: Hypertension*, http://www.nice.org.uk/nicemedia/live/13561/56008/56008.pdf.

NICE (2008) *Clinical Guideline 73: Chronic kidney disease*, http://www.nice.org.uk/CG073.

NICE (2009) *Clinical Guideline 87: Type 2 diabetes*, http://www.nice.org.uk/nicemedia/pdf/CG087NICEGuideline.pdf.

Ruggenenti P, Perna A, Gherardi G *et al.* (1998) Renal function and requirement for dialysis in chronic nephropathy patients on long-term ramipril: REIN follow-up trial. Gruppo Italiano di Studi Epidemiologici in Nefrologia (GISEN). Ramipril Efficacy in Nephropathy. *Lancet* **352**: 1252–6.

Taal M (2011) Predicting renal risk in the general population: Do we have the right formula? *Clin J Am Soc Nephrol* **6**: 1523–5.

UK PD Study.

UK Renal Registry (2009) *Annual Report*, http://www.renalreg.com/Reports/2009.html.

Vivante A, Afek A, Frenkel-Nir Y (2011) Persistent asymptomatic isolated microscopic hematuria in Israeli adolescents and young adults at risk for end-stage renal disease. *JAMA* **306**: 729–36.

CHAPTER 4

Pre-Dialysis Clinics: Preparing for End-Stage Renal Disease

Irene Hadjimichael, Eleri Wood and Katie Vinen

King's College Hospital NHS Foundation Trust, London, UK

OVERVIEW

- Only a small proportion of patients attending general nephrology clinics will eventually progress to stage 5 chronic kidney disease (CKD).

- Up to 25% of patients starting renal replacement therapy do so without being previously known to renal teams. Such 'crash landers' have been shown to have poorer outcomes than those starting dialysis through dedicated pre-dialysis clinics. (See Chapter 13 and Appendix 4).

- Supporting patients through the huge changes associated with end-stage renal failure (ESRF) requires the input of a complex, dedicated multiprofessional team.

- Good education about their condition and their choices (including that provided by other patients) is key to empowering patients to take control of their health.

- Control of risk factors for progression of kidney disease and treatment of the extensive symptom burden associated with stage 5 CKD are important aspects of pre-dialysis clinical management.

- Patients should be given the full range of dialysis choices and supported in making an individual choice most suitable to their health and lifestyle.

- Some older, frailer patients may feel that the burden of dialysis is too great – they should continue to receive specialized care in the maximal supportive care pathway focusing on symptom relief and planning of where and how they would like to be looked after at the end of their life.

- For those in whom it is possible, priority should be given to work up for a pre-emptive living donor transplant but all suitable patients should undergo work up for activation on the cadaveric transplant list.

- The decision for a patient to start dialysis usually reflects a combination of increasing uraemic symptoms and increasingly abnormal biochemistry.

Every year, a small proportion of patients attending general nephrology clinics will progress to the point where clinicians feel that end-stage renal failure (ESRF) is likely within the next year. Dedicated pre-dialysis (or low clearance) clinics (LCCs) have been introduced in the last 15 years to deliver well-organized, patient-focused, multidisciplinary team care to improve their dialysis, transplantation and conservative care outcomes. The team consists of nephrologists, surgeons, nurses, dieticians, counsellors and social workers, who provide holistic care by focusing on correction of chronic kidney disease (CKD) complications, cardiovascular risk management, patient education and early preparation for renal replacement therapy (RRT) or maximal conservative care (Figure 4.1).

For some patients (such as those with a family history of adult polycystic kidney disease who have seen family members reach ESRF), this phase of care is an inevitable and expected progression of their renal journey. For many others, who have previously understood their kidney disease to be relatively minor, this is the first point at which they realize the very significant effect their kidney disease will have on their lifestyle, their employment and their family.

Various studies have demonstrated that early referral to pre-dialysis clinics is associated with:

(i) more favourable patient outcomes including lower morbidity and mortality
(ii) improved education and more active patient participation in the selection of mode of RRT
(iii) reduced urgent initiation of dialysis and hospitalization rates.

Additional benefits include:

(iv) preservation of existing renal function with a delay in the need to initiate RRT
(v) an increased proportion of patients initiating haemodialysis (HD) using a fistula
(vi) better clinical variables at the start of RRT.

The (2004) National Service Framework for Renal Services' guidelines recommend that patients whose estimated glomerular filtration rate (eGFR) is $< 30 \, \text{mL/min}/1.73 \, \text{m}^2$ (CKD stages 4–5) and declining be referred to the pre-dialysis (low clearance) clinic at least a year before RRT is needed. In clinical practice, most nephrologists refer patients to pre-dialysis clinics with a creatinine clearance of $< 15–20 \, \text{mL/min}$ and falling or an expected start of RRT within 6–12 months.

ABC of Kidney Disease, Second edition.
Edited by David Goldsmith, Satish Jayawardene and Penny Ackland.

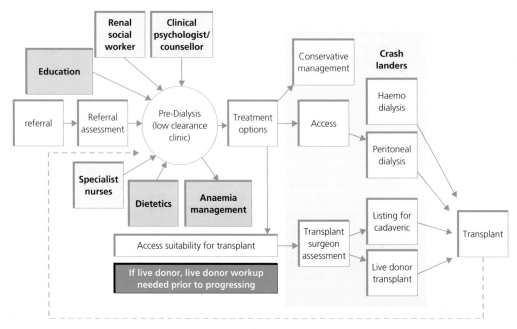

Figure 4.1 Pathway from nephrology to RRT. (*Source:* Adapted from NHS Institute for Innovation and Improvement publication).

In this chapter, the different roles of the pre-dialysis team in providing optimal, high-quality care to patients approaching ESRF will be discussed (Figure 4.1).

Education

Extensive patient education is central to optimal pre-dialysis care and uses various measures (comprehensive and culturally appropriate information booklets, DVDs/CDs, education days and one-to-one visits, Figure 4.2). Patients, families and carers attend multidisciplinary group education days. Education may begin with a basic explanation of where the kidneys are located in the body and what functions they perform, right up to explaining the various medications and treatment options, including dialysis, transplantation and maximal conservative care (see Chapters 9, 10 and 11). Patients are taught how to understand their own blood test results and are given talks on diet and anaemia management in renal failure. Such sessions also give patients the opportunity to meet other patients who may be approaching dialysis or who are already receiving renal replacement therapy, thus facilitating adjustment and normalization of their diagnosis. There is evidence that patients participating in education programmes have improved psychological and social outcomes. All the above measures help to facilitate informed involvement in the decision-making progress and encourage self-management and home dialysis therapies (see Chapter 10), thus allowing patients to take a degree of control over living with a chronic condition. Unfortunately, a small proportion of patients struggle to accept their prognosis and thus refuse or are unable to participate in education sessions or the decision-making process. Varied strategies should be employed to engage patients who are in denial, such as the use of peer supporters and motivational interviewing techniques, but expert communication skills used with persistence, sensitivity and empathy provide the best basis from which to develop trusting constructive relationships with all patients.

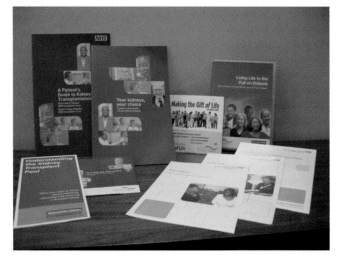

Figure 4.2 Education resources.

Post-dialysis education is also important to 'crash landers' who enter the system as emergencies within 90 days of requiring RRT (and often in immediate need of RRT) and subsequently have poorer outcomes. The pre-dialysis team provide education to this group to lessen the adverse effects and ensure that they are also given the choice to move onto self-care therapies rather than automatically remaining on their initial therapy, which is usually HD.

Preservation of existing renal function and reduction of cardiovascular risk factors

The rate of decline of renal function varies between patients and depends on the cause of the primary disease, race and the presence of exacerbating factors. Cardiovascular morbidity and mortality are significant in patients with stages 4 and 5 CKD.

Table 4.1 Factors for preserving renal function and reducing cardiovascular risk.

Risk factor for progression of CKD or cardiovascular risk	Intervention	Target value (where applicable)
Hypertension	Control with salt and fluid restriction, exercise, antihypertensive medications	< 140/90 mmHg in patients with CKD < 130/80 mmHg in patients with CKD and diabetes or proteinuria $\geq$ 1 g
Hyperglycaemia	Dietary advice, weight reduction, oral hypoglycaemics and insulin	HbA1c < 7.5% without frequent hypoglycaemic attacks
Dyslipidaemia	Dietary advice, statins	Total cholesterol < 4 mmol/L for secondary prevention and diabetes Total cholesterol < 5 mmol/L for others
Acidosis	Supplementation with oral bicarbonate	Maintain serum bicarbonate levels over or at 22 mmol/L
Minimize proteinuria	ACE inhibition, angiotensin receptor inhibition	Urinary protein levels of < 0.5 g/24 h
Nephrotoxic drugs	Avoid NSAIDs, trimethoprim and radiological or angiographic contrast media.	

ACE, angiotensin converting enzyme; NSAIDs, nonsteroidal anti-inflammatory drugs.

In the pre-dialysis clinic, many factors are addressed to preserve existing renal function and to reduce cardiovascular risk (Table 4.1).

All patients should also be encouraged to adopt a healthy lifestyle with cessation of smoking, increased exercise and a target BMI of 20–25. Careful liaison with colleagues in urology, cardiology, vascular surgery and radiology is needed to ensure avoidance/minimization of radiological contrast and prompt treatment of urinary obstruction. Additional measures to reduce adverse cardiovascular outcomes include antiplatelet therapy (if estimated 10-year risk of cardiovascular disease > 20%), treating anaemia (which can lead to left ventricular hypertrophy) and treating mineral bone disorders.

Addressing complications of chronic kidney disease

Management of fluid overload

Salt and fluid overload is common and leads to hypertension, peripheral and pulmonary oedema (Figure 4.3). Measures to control fluid overload include salt and fluid intake restriction (1–1.5 L/day) and the use of diuretics (furosemide, metolazone) while monitoring the patient's weight, blood pressure (BP), electrolyte and renal function to avoid over-diuresis.

Management of hyperkalaemia and metabolic acidosis

Hyperkalaemia is a potentially life-threatening condition. Out-patient preventative measures include avoidance of potassium rich foods (Figure 4.4, see Further reading), loop diuretics, withdrawal of unnecessary contributory drugs (spironolactone, frumil, NSAIDs, beta blockers) and dose reduction or cessation of ACE inhibitors or angiotensin receptor blockers. Correction of acidosis with sodium bicarbonate not only helps hyperkalaemia but may also prevent inflammation, malnutrition, increased bone resorption and impaired mineralization, muscle weakness and fatigue.

Management of uraemic symptoms

The uraemic syndrome consists of pruritus, restless legs, muscle cramps, anorexia, nausea, vomiting, tiredness, altered taste sensation, poor concentration, changes to sleep patterns and sexual dysfunction. These symptoms are often hard to treat and cause considerable distress. Treatments including gabapentin (neuropathy), clonazepam (restless legs), quinine sulphate and tonic water (cramps), antihistamines, gabapentin and topical creams

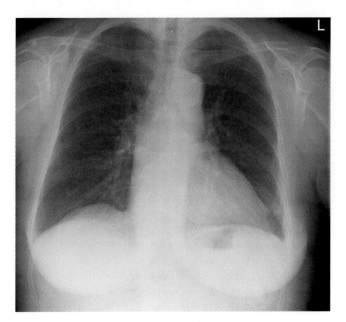

Figure 4.3 Chest x-ray illustrating fluid overload pulmonary oedema.

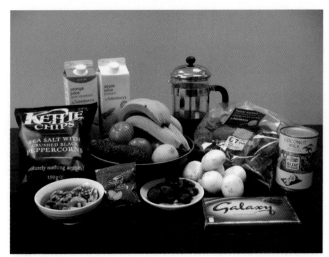

Figure 4.4 High potassium foods.

(pruritus) and anti-emetics and proton pumps inhibitors (nausea and vomiting) may provide relief. While significant symptoms have often been seen as an indication to start RRT, more recent research in fact suggests that many patients retain many symptoms despite starting dialysis treatment.

Management of anaemia

Anaemia is common in ESRF and results from a combination of deficiencies in erythropoietin (EPO), iron, B12 and folate, and reduced red cell survival due to uraemia, hyperparathyroidism and chronic inflammation. Severe anaemia contributes to left ventricular hypertrophy and systolic dysfunction, fatigue, impaired cognitive function and lower quality of life (poor sleep, sexual dysfunction).

Management of anaemia first involves exclusion of other non-renal causes such as gastrointestinal (GI) bleeding. This is followed by replenishing iron stores by intravenous iron if the patient is deficient, and then commencing erythropoiesis-stimulating agent (ESA) therapy. During treatment, the patient's BP and blood results are monitored to achieve the targets set by the National Institute for Health and Clinical Excellence (NICE): haemoglobin of 10.0–11.5 g/dL, serum ferritin 200–500 μg/L, and either transferrin saturation > 20% or % hypochromic red cells < 6%. For more information on management of anaemia in CKD, see Chapter 5.

Management of chronic kidney disease-mineral and bone disorder (CKD-MBD)

CKD-MBD is a systemic disorder manifested by abnormalities in bone and mineral metabolism and extra-skeletal calcification. It can lead to pruritus, soft tissue calcification, fractures, bone and joint pain, vascular calcification and cardiovascular disease, and even premature death. It results from decreased production (conversion) of 1,25-dihydroxyvitamin D3 (calcitriol) in the failing kidney, leading to deranged plasma calcium concentration, hyperparathyroidism and phosphate retention. While an initial rise in parathyroid hormone level is homeostatic, resulting in a lowering of serum phosphate levels and a rise in calcium levels, persistent secondary hyperparathyroidism together with high phosphate values and deranged calcium values can lead to renal bone disease. Its treatment at relatively early stages of CKD is not based on a wealth of evidence, but should focus on management of phosphate intake in the diet, and by judicious use of vitamin D compounds. Guidance on these matters has been provided by the UK Renal Association for patients with CKD stages CKD 3-5 (not yet on dialysis) (Table 4.2). These cases can be complex so detailed feedback and advice from the local renal unit is encouraged.

Planning for end-stage renal failure

Patients should be provided with sufficient time and information to allow them to make an informed and timely decision regarding their preferred ESRF therapy pathway. The decision between transplantation, HD and peritoneal dialysis (PD), and conservative care

Table 4.2 Renal Association guidelines for CKD-MBD.

Target	Management
Phosphate: maintain between 0.9 and 1.5 mmol/L	Dietary phosphate restriction (800 mg/day) Phosphate binding medication with meals
Corrected calcium: within normal reference range	Vitamin D supplementation with one alpha calcidol
	Manipulation of calcium intake through selective use of non-calcium or calcium-based phosphate binders
PTH: treat if PTH levels are progressively rising and remain high despite correction of modifiable factors	It is not normally necessary to measure PTH at all in CKD stage 3a patients unless there are marked abnormalities in plasma calcium or phosphate concentrations. PTH should be measured annually (either in secondary or in primary care) in CKD stage 3b. Measurement and management of CKD-MBD in CKD stage 4 patients should be discussed with the local kidney specialists. Measurement of 25(OH) vitamin D concentrations is desirable for those with CKD stage 3a and 3b and some evidence of associated bone disease, e.g. osteoporosis. Repletion however should be decided on carefully, plasma calcium and phosphate concentrations monitored regularly, and discussed with the local kidney specialists.

PTH, Parathyroid Hormone.

should not be influenced by either clinicians' prejudice or local resources.

Transplant education and work-up

Renal transplantation (where clinically appropriate) is the ideal form of RRT in terms of patient survival, quality of life and cost-effectiveness. These benefits are increased if the transplant is performed pre-emptively (i.e. before patients are established on dialysis) and thus patients are encouraged to seek a live donor or are placed on the national transplant waiting list up to six months ahead of their anticipated dialysis start date. Strict listing criteria only allow activation of patients who are fit to undergo surgery and long-term immunosuppression.

Transplant coordinators work in parallel with the main low clearance clinic to help ensure patients are suitably counselled and prepared. Investigations for both recipients and donors can take several months and include ECG, CXR, virology, tissue typing, cardiac testing, carotid and leg arterial dopplers and post-micturition bladder ultrasound.

For more information on renal transplantation please refer to Chapter 11.

Dialysis choice

After receiving extensive education, patients make a choice between PD (always performed at home) and HD (usually performed at hospital with a small percentage haemodialysing in their own home).

There are no adequate randomized controlled trials comparing outcomes of PD with HD, or of home- versus centre-based therapies. The optimal treatment for a given patient can be affected by coexistent medical conditions (such as availability of good vessels for fistula creation or previous abdominal surgery preventing peritoneal dialysis) but is generally determined by their desire and ability to deliver their own dialysis and lifestyle factors (such as a desire to continue working or travelling extensively often favouring PD). NICE commissioned a systematic review of home- versus hospital- or satellite-based HD, which, despite the lack of grade 1 evidence, concluded that the home therapy offered advantages to patients in terms of quality of life, flexibility, reduced travel, improved survival and was cost-effective to the NHS See Chapters 10, 11, and 13.

Creation of dialysis access

There is strong evidence that permanent dialysis access should be established early to reduce the risk of morbidity and mortality. Where there is a preference for HD, doppler ultrasound vessel mapping of the non-dominant arm is performed and venepuncture is avoided in the arms. Early surgery is important as an arteriovenous fistula (AVF) takes 4–8 weeks to mature to being usable, and ideally should occur at least six months before dialysis commences. Where there is preference for PD and provided there are no medical (*previous major abdominal surgery, intra-abdominal adhesions, abdominal wall stoma, intestinal disease, severe respiratory disease, impaired manual dexterity or vision as seen in some diabetics*) or social (*housing, poor support*) contraindications, a Tenckhoff catheter can be inserted into the abdomen either under local or general anaesthetic. It can be used within 24 hours if urgent dialysis is required but ideally should be rested for 3–4 weeks.

For more information on dialysis, see Chapter 10.

Hepatitis B vaccination

All patients who are likely to require RRT should be vaccinated against Hepatitis B to reduce the possibility of cross infection from this blood-based treatment. Vaccination in the early stages of CKD has a better seroconversion rate to full immunity than late vaccination does.

Conservative care

Recent studies show that dialysis may not improve quantity or quality of life in older, dependent patients with extensive comorbidities. This is important as much of the recent growth in numbers reaching stage 5 kidney disease has been in the over-70s. Some of these patients opt for conservative care after discussion with their family and the multidisciplinary team. The conservative approach aims to provide all aspects of active clinical care (protecting remaining renal function, managing complications and symptoms of CKD), with the exception of RRT. In addition, and in liaison with community and palliative care services, patients receive advanced care planning establishing how and where they would like to be looked after as they become frailer. Such patients often have a significantly better quality of life with fewer hospital admissions and are more likely to die at home rather than in hospital compared to equivalent patients on dialysis.

For more information on conservative treatment for patients with CKD, please refer to Chapter 9.

Additional care given in low clearance clinics

Dietetic support

Dieticians play a vital role in the care of patients with ESRF by taking into account the patient's weight, lifestyle, diet and blood results, and providing individual culturally specific advice (for instance where it relates to an Afro-Caribbean or Asian diet) (Box 4.1).

Box 4.1 Role of dietician in low clearance clinics

Medical history and nutritional assessment (food diary, malnutrition screening, review of GI symptoms and weight changes over previous six months)
Advice for weight loss > 10% in past 3–6 months
Advice for high BMI
Advice for diabetics with high HbA1C/sugars
Advice on a low phosphate diet and correct use of phosphate binders (to be taken with food or in 15 minutes prior to food)
Advice on a low potassium diet (see Further Reading)
Advice on salt (< 6 g per day) and fluid restriction (< 1.5 L/day)

Social and psychological support

Many patients experience the pre-dialysis phase as stressful as they face changes in employment, social status, ability to obtain insurance and mortgages and ability to travel. The multidisciplinary team supports patients on their road to acceptance and at all times endeavours to promote self-management.

Social workers and counsellors are invaluable and can offer practical help, advice and support (Box 4.2). Many units now also

---

Box 4.2 Role of social worker and counsellor in low clearance clinics

Role of social worker

Advice on eligibility for benefits and social support
Advice on housing options (particularly where changes to housing may allow the use of a home dialysis therapy)
Advice about employment rights
Advice about legal issues such as immigration issues, power of attorney or preparation of a will

Role of counsellor in low clearance clinics

Advice on coming to terms with living with a chronic disease
Help with anxiety and depression
Help in managing strains on work and family life
Counselling on managing change of body image issues (e.g. after insertion of a Tenckhoff catheter)
Help to relatives of patients with loss and bereavement

offer peer support programmes where newer patients meet with trained experienced patients providing practical and emotional support as well as further education about living with renal disease.

Decision to start dialysis

The optimal timing of initiating renal replacement therapy in patients with CKD remains controversial. One study has demonstrated that survival and adverse event rates were similar between a group of patients randomized to begin dialysis at an eGFR of 10.0–14.0 mL/min (early start) and a group randomized to start at an eGFR of 5.0–7.0 mL/min (late start). See Chapter 10.

In clinical practice, there is considerable variation in the timing of initiation of maintenance dialysis. The European Best Practice Guidelines recommend that RRT should commence when a patient with an eGFR < 15 mL/min/1.73 m^2 has symptoms or signs of uraemia, fluid overload, severe hyperkalaemia or malnutrition in spite of medical therapy or before eGFR has fallen below 6 mL/min/1.73 m^2 in an asymptomatic patient. In the majority of patients a combination of symptoms and biochemical parameters will contribute to their start date, with most patients starting PD with a GFR of 12–14 mL/min and most starting HD with a GFR of 8–12 mL/minute.

Further reading

Department of Health (2004) *The National Service Framework for Renal Services. Part One: Dialysis and Transplantation.* Department of Health, London.

Goovaerts T, Jadoul M, Goffin E (2005) Influence of a pre-dialysis education programme on the mode of RRT. *Nephrol Dial Transplant* 20: 1842–7.

Jafar TH, Stark TPC, Schmid CH et al. (2003) Progression of chronic kidney disease: The role of blood pressure control, proteinuria, and ACE inhibition: A patient-level meta-analysis. *Ann Intern Med* 139: 244–52.

Khan SS, Xue JL, Kazmi WH et al. (2005) Does predialysis nephrology care influence patient survival after initiation of dialysis? *Kidney Int* 67: 1038–46.

Morton RL, Tong A, Howard K et al. (2010) The views of patients and carers in treatment decision making for chronic kidney disease: Systematic review and thematic synthesis of qualitative studies. *BMJ* 340: 112.

National Kidney Foundation. (2012) High potassium food table, http://www.kidney.org/atoz/content/potassium.cfm.

NHS Institute for Innovation and Improvement (2008) Focus on: Preparing for End-Stage Renal Disease, http://www.institute.nhs.uk/quality_and_value/high_volume_care/focus_on%3A_renal.html

NHS R&D HTA Programme (2002) Systematic review of the effectiveness and cost-effectiveness of home versus hospital or satellite unit haemodialysis for people with end stage renal failure, http://www.nice.org.uk/nicemedia/pdf/HvH_Assessment_report.pdf.

Owen JE, Walker RJ, Edgell L et al. (2006) Implementation of a pre-dialysis clinical pathway for patients with chronic kidney disease. *Int J Qual Health Care* 18(2): 145–51.

Rayner HC, Besarab A, Brown WW et al. (2004) Vascular access results from the Dialysis Outcomes and Practice Patterns Study (DOPPS): Performance against Kidney Disease Outcomes Quality Initiative (K/DOQI) Clinical Practice Guidelines. *Am J Kidney Dis* 44(suppl. 3): 22–6.

Renal Association (2011) Planning, Initiating and Withdrawal of Renal Replacement Therapy, http://www.renal.org/clinical/guidelinessection/RenalReplacementTherapy.aspx

UK Renal Registry (2009) *Annual Report*, http://www.renalreg.com/Reports/2009.html.

Yaqoob MM (2009) Bicarbonate supplementation slows progression of CKD and improves nutritional status. *J Am Soc Nephrol* 20(9): 1869–70.

CHAPTER 5

Anaemia Management in Chronic Kidney Disease

Penny Ackland

Nunhead Surgery, Nunhead Grove, South East London, UK

OVERVIEW

- The overall incidence of anaemia in chronic kidney disease (CKD) stages 3, 4 and 5 is around 12%.
- Anaemia of CKD can start to develop when the estimated glomerular filtration rate (eGFR) <60 mL/min/1.73 m^2, and its prevalence and severity increases as kidney function declines.
- If severe iron deficiency is present (e.g. serum ferritin <30 mcg/L), then it is important to consider blood loss as a possible cause of the anaemia.
- Investigation and treatment of anaemia should be considered if the haemoglobin (Hb) is <11 g/dL or symptoms attributable to anaemia develop.
- Absolute iron-deficiency anaemia is diagnosed when serum ferritin is <100 µg/L in CKD stage 5, and should be considered when serum ferritin is <100 µg/L in CKD stages 3 and 4.
- Functional iron deficiency is defined by a serum ferritin level >100 µg/L and either the hypochromic red cells (HRC) is >6% or the transferrin saturation (TSAT) is <20%.
- The iron correction should aim to maintain the ferritin >200 µg/L, TSAT >20%, and % HRC <6% (unless the ferritin >800 µg/L).
- The iron dose should be reviewed when the ferritin reaches 500 µg/L (it should not rise above 800 µg/L).
- Treatment with erythropoiesis-stimulating agent (ESA) therapy is not generally recommended until the Hb is likely to fall below 10 g/dL – typically the aspirational range of ESA-corrected Hb should lie between 10 and 12 g/dL for adults.

Prevalence and impact of anaemia of chronic kidney disease

Anaemia in CKD affects around 100 000 people in the United Kingdom (NICE 2011) and contributes significantly to the heavy symptom burden of CKD. It becomes more prevalent the more advanced the stage of CKD (1% of people with an eGFR of 60 mL/min, 9% of people with an eGFR of 30 mL/min and 33%

of people with an eGFR of 15 mL/min are anaemic). The overall incidence of anaemia in CKD stages 3 to 5 is 12%. Not only can its presence have a major negative impact on the quality of life and physical capacity of the individual, but it may also increase cardiac output and left ventricular hypertrophy (London 2003) Other possible adverse effects of anaemia are (NICE 2011):

- increased bleeding time/impaired platelet function
- reduced cognition and concentration
- reduced libido
- reduced immune responsiveness.

Causes

The anaemia of CKD is normochromic and normocytic in nature. The cause is multifactorial, but by far the main contribution is the reduced erythropoietic activity caused by iron deficiency or erythropoietin deficiency, or both. Other minor causes may also contribute to the anaemia of CKD.

Erythropoietin is a hormone produced by the peritubular cells in the kidney, which is critically involved in the manufacture of red blood cells in the bone marrow. Iron is an essential mineral for the production of haem, the oxygen-carrying component of Hb. Iron deficiency may be *functional* (when body iron stores may be normal or increased but there is a failure of iron delivery to the bone marrow) or *absolute* (when body iron stores are exhausted) (NICE 2011). The latter condition occurs, in part, because of impaired absorption of iron from the gastrointestinal (GI) tract in uraemia and partly due to increased iron losses as a result of platelet dysfunction associated with, for example, uraemia or aspirin therapy. Furthermore, dialysis may exacerbate increased iron deficiency by the trapping of red cells in the dialyser.

As a result of the inflammation that is associated with CKD (uraemia is now recognized to be a chronic inflammatory state), the serum ferritin is often raised, and diagnostic values need to be interpreted differently from those in patients without this disease: iron-deficiency anaemia is diagnosed when serum ferritin is <100 µg/L in CKD stage 5 and should be considered when serum ferritin is <100 µg/L in CKD stages 3 and 4.

Laboratory parameters, other than serum ferritin, which may be used for detecting iron deficiency, include the transferrin

---

ABC of Kidney Disease, Second edition.
Edited by David Goldsmith, Satish Jayawardene and Penny Ackland.

saturation[1] (TSAT) and the percentage of hypochromic red cells (HRC). Even when the serum ferritin is greater than 100 mcg/L, functional iron deficiency may still be present if the transferrin saturation is <20% or the percentage of HRC is >6%.

Measurement of erythropoietin levels is usually unhelpful in the diagnosis of CKD anaemia, and should not be routinely considered for the investigation of this condition (NICE 2011).

Previous management practices

Prior to 1990, severe anaemia of CKD was generally treated with top-up blood transfusions every 2–4 weeks. In many cases, this led to iron overload, infections, allergic reactions and increased sensitization to human leukocyte antigens with consequential difficulties if transplantation was considered. The management of anaemia related to CKD was revolutionized by the introduction of recombinant human erythropoietin in the late 1980s (National Clinical Guideline Centre 2011). Since then, longer-acting erythropoietin analogues have become available, and this class of drugs is known as the erythropoiesis-stimulating agents (ESAs), which have allowed earlier and more sustained treatment of the anaemia.

In order to provide evidence for clinical decision-making on the management of anaemia, several randomized controlled trials have been conducted (Besarab et al. 1998; Drüeke et al. 2006; Singh et al. 2006; Pfeffer et al. 2009). The CREATE (Cardiovascular Risk Reduction by Early Anemia Treatment with Epoetin Beta) and the CHOIR (Correction of Hemoglobin and Outcomes in Renal Insufficiency) studies (Drüeke et al. 2006; Singh et al. 2006) stirred up some unease about the safety of ESA therapy. However, it was the TREAT (Trial to Reduce Cardiovascular Events with Aranesp Therapy) study (Pfeffer et al. 2009) that raised more definitive concerns regarding the safety of using ESA therapy to deliberately target Hb concentrations of 13 g/dL or above.

The TREAT study recruited over 4000 patients, who were randomized into one of two arms:

- an 'active' arm targeting an Hb of around 13 g/dL with ESA therapy;
- a 'control' arm receiving placebo treatment with 'rescue' ESA therapy if the Hb fell below 9 g/dL (this placebo group started with a level of about 10.5 g/dL and drifted up to around 11 g/dL at the end of the study).

Although there were no significant differences in the overall composite endpoint of death, heart failure, myocardial infarction and stroke, there were a number of pertinent safety outcomes, which caused concern:

- stroke (risk was doubled compared with the control group);

---

[1]The total iron-binding capacity measures the blood's capacity to bind iron with transferrin, a glycoprotein that binds iron very tightly but reversibly. The *transferrin saturation* is the ratio of serum iron and total iron-binding capacity multiplied by 100. Of the transferrin that is available to bind iron, the transferrin saturation tells a clinician how much serum iron is actually bound.

- venous thromboembolism (risk was almost doubled compared with the control group);
- arterial thromboembolism (slightly higher rate compared with the control group);
- >10-fold risk of cancer-related mortality in patients who had experienced a previous malignancy.

Post-hoc analyses of these trials suggest that the risk from ESAs is greatest in patients who are resistant to this particular type of therapy and need larger quantities of ESAs to normalize Hb levels (Szczech et al. 2008; Solomon et al. 2010).

As a consequence, the use of ESAs to correct Hb to normal levels (generally considered to lie between 12 and 14 g/dL in women, and 13 and 16 g/dL in men) is not usually recommended in patients with CKD-related anaemia.

Current management

In order to optimize the management of anaemia of CKD, it may be helpful to adopt a step-wise approach.

1. Patients with anaemia should be highlighted

Within general practice this should be done when setting up the CKD register as part of the Quality and Outcomes Framework (QOF) (British Medical Association 2009). The overall incidence of anaemia in CKD stages 3, 4 and 5 is around 12% (National Clinical Guideline Centre 2011).

2. Other causes of anaemia should be excluded (see Box 5.1)

Anaemia of CKD can start to develop when the eGFR <60 mL/min/1.73 m^2, and its prevalence and severity increases as kidney function declines. NICE advises that, 'an estimated glomerular filtration rate of less than 60 mL/min/1.73 m^2 should trigger investigation into whether anaemia is due to CKD' (NICE 2011).

> Box 5.1 **Other possible causes of anaemia in chronic kidney disease**
>
> - Chronic blood loss
> - Iron deficiency
> - Vitamin B$_{12}$ or folate deficiency
> - Hypothyroidism
> - Chronic infection or inflammation
> - Hyperparathyroidism
> - Malignancy
> - Haemolysis
> - Bone marrow infiltration
> - Pure red cell aplasia

If severe iron deficiency is present (e.g. serum ferritin <30 mcg/L), then it is important to consider blood loss as a possible cause of the anaemia.

3. Investigation and treatment of anaemia attributable to CKD should be considered if the Hb is <11 g/dL

(or ≤10.5 g/dL if the patient is aged <2 years), or if the patient develops symptoms attributable to anaemia (e.g. tiredness, shortness of breath, lethargy and palpitations) (NICE 2011). (See Appendix 1, Table A1.2).

(i) **Iron status should be determined** (whether functional or absolute deficiency) (NICE 2011).

Serum ferritin is often raised in CKD; the diagnostic cut-off value should be interpreted differently from that in patients without CKD:

- Absolute iron-deficiency anaemia is diagnosed when serum ferritin is <100 μg/L in CKD stage 5, and should be considered when serum ferritin is <100 μg/L in CKD stages 3 and 4;
- Functional iron deficiency is defined by a serum ferritin level >100 μg/L and either the HRC is >6% or TSAT is <20%.

(ii) **Iron deficiency should be treated, and iron status optimized** (NICE 2011).

Oral iron frequently causes GI side-effects. It is poorly absorbed in uraemic patients. This is now known to be due to increased levels of a recently discovered peptide hormone called hepcidin, which is the master regulator of iron metabolism in the body, and which is upregulated in chronic inflammatory states such as CKD. High hepcidin levels inhibit both the absorption of dietary iron and oral iron supplements from the duodenum. Intravenous iron should be used to treat both functional iron deficiency and patients who do not respond to (or tolerate) oral iron. Iron status should be optimized before deciding whether to use ESAs in non-dialysis patients.

(iii) **The iron correction should aim to maintain the ferritin > 200 μg/L, TSAT > 20%, and % HRC < 6% (unless the ferritin > 800 μg/L)** (NICE 2011).

(iv) **The iron dose should be reviewed when the ferritin reaches 500 μg/L (it should not rise above 800 μg/L)** (NICE 2011).

4. One should consider referral to secondary care for ESA therapy if:

- patients are likely to benefit in quality of life and physical function;
- comorbidities and prognosis are unlikely to negate the benefit of correcting the anaemia with ESAs;
- there is uncertainty regarding the benefit:risk ratio of ESA therapy (a trial of the therapy may be warranted).

(i) **Treatment with ESA therapy is not generally recommended until the Hb is likely to fall below 10 g/dL – typically the aspirational range of ESA-corrected Hb should lie between 10 and 12 g/dL for adults** (or between 9.5 and 11.5 g/dL for children younger than 2 years of age) (NICE 2011).

The following factors should be taken into account when determining individual aspirational Hb ranges for people with anaemia of CKD:

- patient preferences
- symptoms and comorbidities
- the required treatment.

Hb should be kept within this aspirational range; healthcare professionals should not wait until Hb levels are outside this range before adjusting treatment (e.g. action should be taken when Hb levels are within 0.5 g/dL of the range's limits) (NICE 2011).

It is important to be aware that iron demand increases with both ESA initiation and dialysis.

5. Age alone should not be a determinant for treating anaemia of CKD

(NICE 2011).

6. In patients who are showing a poor response to treatment, one should:

- evaluate concordance;
- measure reticulocyte count – if high, consider blood loss and haemolysis;
- exclude other causes of anaemia (Box 5.1);
- exclude intercurrent illness;
- exclude chronic blood loss;
- consider bone marrow examination.

The role of care in the community

Erythropoietin therapy tends not to be managed within the primary care setting. However, in the current climate of cost rationing, provision of care closer to home and the increasing prevalence of CKD, it is likely that management of patients with anaemia related to CKD will be under the domain of general practice. Some CKD patients with advanced renal impairment may be directed down a palliative care pathway if dialysis is not appropriate and, if cared for at home, may benefit from iron supplementation and ESA therapy provided via the community.

Recent trial evidence has led to a paradigm shift in anaemia management in people with CKD, now recommending that the correction of anaemia with ESAs should not usually occur until the Hb level is likely to fall below 10 g/dL. Hence, there is scope for increasing the management of anaemia within primary care, particularly if intravenous iron can be delivered in a primary care setting. When considering ESA therapy, it is clear that a carefully considered balance is needed between the benefits (such as reduced red cell transfusions and increased quality of life) and potential harm (from increased risk of stroke and venous thromboembolism, and possible exacerbation of malignancy) of this treatment. Individualization of therapy has become more important than ever, with increased recognition of factors affecting the benefit:risk ratio of treatment.

References

Besarab A, Bolton W, Browne J et al. (1998) The effects of normal as compared with low hematocrit values in patients with cardiac disease who are receiving hemodialysis and epoetin. *N Engl J Med* **339**(9): 584–90.

British Medical Association (2009) *Quality and Outcomes Framework Guidance for GMS Contract, 2009/10: Delivering investment in general practice.* BMA, London. Available at: http://www.bma.org.uk/employment andcontracts/independent_contractors/quality_outcomes_framework.

Drüeke T, Locatelli F, Clyne N et al. (2006) CREATE Investigators: Normalization of haemoglobin level in patients with chronic kidney disease and anemia. *N Engl J Med* **355**(20): 2071–84.

London G (2003) Cardiovascular disease in chronic renal failure: Pathophysiologic aspects. *Semin Dial* **16**(2): 85–94.

NICE (2011) *Anaemia management in chronic kidney disease: Rapid update 2011.* http://www.nice.org.uk/CG114.

NICE (2011) *Clinical Guideline 114: Anaemia Management in People with Chronic Kidney Disease.* http://www.nice.org.uk/CG114.

Pfeffer M, Burdmann E, Chen C et al. (2009) TREAT Investigators: A trial of darbepoetin alfa in type 2 diabetes and chronic kidney disease. *N Engl J Med* **361**(21): 2019–2032.

Singh A, Szczech L, Tang K et al. (2006) CHOIR Investigators 2006. Correction of anemia with epoetin alfa in chronic kidney disease. *N Engl J Med* **355**(20): 2085–98.

Solomon S, Uno H, Lewis E et al. (2010) Erythropoietic response and outcomes in kidney disease and type 2 diabetes. *N Engl J Med* **363**(12): 1146–55.

Szczech L, Barnhart H, Inrig J et al. (2008) Secondary analysis of the CHOIR trial epoetin-alpha dose and achieved hemoglobin outcomes. *Kidney Int* **74**(6): 791–8.

CHAPTER 6

Urinary Tract Infections, Renal Stones, Renal Cysts and Tumours and Pregnancy in Chronic Kidney Disease

David Goldsmith

King's College London, London, UK

OVERVIEW

- Dysuria is usually urinary tract infection-related, but it can be due to urethritis (e.g. chlamydia, herpes) or vaginitis (e.g. *Trichomonas* spp).

- Asymptomatic bacteriuria does not generally need treatment except in pregnancy.

- Pyelonephritis and renal abscesses are potentially life threatening.

- Acute pyelonephritis is suggested by fever, chills, flank pain, raised CRP (C-reactive protein) and white cell count.

- Kidney stones may vary from being asymptomatic, if tiny, to causing colicky loin (often radiating to groin) pain with visible haematuria. The pain may be so severe as to cause vomiting. The risk of infection and obstruction with such cases warrants urgent investigation.

- Kidney stones form in urine that is supersaturated with the chemical constituents. The main types are calcium oxalate, calcium phosphate struvite, urate and cystine.

- Calcium stones are exacerbated by loop diuretics, vitamin D, antacids and steroids, while uric acid stones can be exacerbated by salicylates and are more common in people of Middle Eastern and Mediterranean origin.

- With increased access to renal/abdominal ultrasound and CT scanning, more renal cysts and masses are being discovered incidentally. Any solid renal mass > 3 cm should be regarded as potentially malignant and considered for removal.

- Fertility declines with advancing chronic kidney disease (CKD), pregnancy being very unusual while on dialysis. Successful renal transplantation has a good chance of restoring fertility.

Urinary tract infections in adults

Acute uncomplicated urinary tract infections (UTIs) are one of the most common medical conditions. Their incidence depends on gender, age, sexual activity and predisposing factors (e.g. urological, anatomical or functional abnormalities, pregnancy, foreign bodies, immunosuppression, host/mucosal immune defences). In sexually active younger women the incidence of cystitis is 0.5 per person per year, whereas in adult men aged less than 50 years it is 5–8 episodes per 10 000 men annually. Infections occur when uropathogens (e.g. *Escherichia coli*) present in rectal flora enter the urinary tract via the urethra. More rarely, UTIs occur by haematogenous spread.

Women with uncomplicated UTIs generally present with dysuria, frequency, urgency and suprapubic pain. Dysuria itself of course can be UTI-related, but can be due to urethritis (e.g. chlamydia, herpes) or vaginitis (*Trichomonas* spp).

In this setting *E. coli* is typically resistant to amoxicillin, and increasing resistance is now being seen to trimethoprim and cotrimoxazole. Trimethoprim is the best first-line option, but it is imperative to be aware of local communities' antibiotic resistance patterns and local hospital/community guidelines. Three-day oral antibiotic courses are preferred (single-dose strategies are less effective, but have fewer side-effects). Recurrent episodes are usually due to incomplete eradication rather than reinfection. Women with recurrent cystitis can opt to try altering certain behavioural risk factors (e.g. voiding post-coitus, increasing fluid intake). Cranberry/lingonberry juice (> 200 mL/day) can help prevent some UTIs. Antibiotic prophylaxis either given regularly (e.g. 100 mg trimethoprim or cephalexin 250 mg nocte), or as a stat post-coital dose, might be a highly effective intervention. If given regularly, rotating the antibiotics every 6 to 12 weeks may reduce the risk of resistance.

Indwelling urinary catheters are the main reason for hospital acquired complex urinary tract infections. Such UTIs are the commonest cause of gram-negative bacteraemias.

Asymptomatic bacteriuria is defined as the presence of two separate clean-voided urine specimens with > 10^5 bacteria/mL of voided urine without symptoms. Five per cent of premenopausal women, and far fewer men, have this. Over the age of 65, around 10% of men and 20% of women have asymptomatic bacteriuria. In pregnancy asymptomatic bacteriuria should be treated to avoid the risk of progression to acute pyelonephritis. Antibiotic sensitivity should be obtained first. Unless there is bacterial resistance, amoxicillin is now generally used first-line (or either nitrofurantoin or a cephalosporin such as cephalexin if penicillin-allergic). Nitrofurantoin should be avoided at term since it can cause anaemia in the newborn, and trimethoprim, being a folate antagonist, should particularly be avoided in the first trimester.

Aetiological agents are typically *E. coli* (75–90%) and *S. saprophyticus* (coagulase-negative staphylococcus; 10–20%). *Proteus* spp,

ABC of Kidney Disease, Second edition.
Edited by David Goldsmith, Satish Jayawardene and Penny Ackland.
© 2013 John Wiley & Sons, Ltd. Published 2013 by John Wiley & Sons, Ltd.

Klebsiella spp and *Enterobacter* spp are also important, though much more rare.

Acute pyelonephritis is suggested by fever, chills, flank pain, raised C-reactive protein (CRP) and white cell count. Cystitis symptoms are present too. White cells in the urine are ubiquitous unless the infected kidney is also obstructed (e.g. ureteric stone). The kidney is inflamed and oedematous. Parenteral or oral therapy can be chosen, depending on the severity of the infection and other patient-related factors; most cases are dealt with by hospital admission. Fourteen-day courses of potent antibiotics are indicated (e.g. cefuroxime, ciprofloxacin).

Infections that have been caused by the presence of a foreign body, e.g. a urinary catheter, or a ureteric stent, may not improve, or may relapse very early, unless that foreign body is removed, or changed.

Renal abscess is a rare event, e.g. 1–10 per 10 000 hospital admissions. The clinical presentation can be fulminant or indolent. Abscesses can be corticomedullary, peri-renal or cortical (e.g. renal carbuncle in the renal cortex due to *S. aureus*). *Papillary necrosis* is also a rare event, caused by hypoxia in the renal medulla, whose risk factors include age, sickle cell disease or trait (and other haemoglobinopathies), diabetes, analgesic abuse and dehydration. Papillary necrosis can cause renal obstruction if the sloughed papillary nubbin lodges in the ureter. *Emphysematous pyelonephritis* is a rare, fulminant necrotizing variant of acute pyelonephritis, often in diabetic patients, and with gas-forming *E. coli, K. pneumoniae, P. mirabilis*; septic peri-nephric haematomata are a complication. *Xanthogranulomatous pyelonephritis* is an even rarer but severe chronic renal infection associated with urinary obstruction. A portion of renal parenchyma is replaced by a dense cellular infiltrate of lipid-laden macrophages; this process can extend outside the kidney. The offending organisms are usually *E. coli* or *S. aureus*.

Kidney stones (nephrolithiasis)

Here, we will discuss only kidney stones (as opposed to stones that form in the bladder or ureter). The main types of renal stone are calcium oxalate, calcium phosphate struvite, urate and cystine. Figures 6.1 and 6.2 shows some renal stones.

Kidney stones can vary from tiny, microscopic deposits with no symptoms to large staghorn calculi filling up the renal pelvis and causing pain, infection and obstruction. Box 6.1 lists the clinical presentation of kidney stone disease; its severity depends on the stone type, rate of formation, size and location.

Box 6.1 **Clinical presentation of kidney stone disease**

- Pain (loin to groin, waves, severe)
- Visible haematuria
- Non-visible haematuria
- Infection
- Obstruction

Kidney stones are common in industrialized countries, with a peak age of onset in the third decade, and an annual incidence

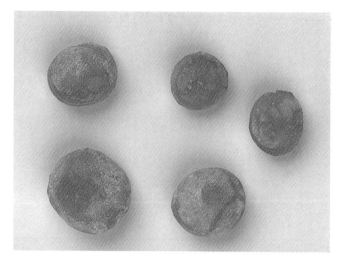

Figure 6.1 Renal stones.

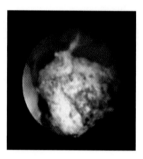

Figure 6.2 Stone obstruction of a ureter (seen at ureterscopy). (*Source:* Reproduced with permission from *ABC of Urology*, Blackwell Publishing Ltd.)

of about 1 in 1000 people. Factors that determine prevalence include age, race, geography and gender. In the Middle East and Mediterranean countries, uric acid stones can be > 50% of all stones, whereas in the United Kingdom they are < 5%. Stone formation can be associated with many different medications: calcium stones with loop diuretics, vitamin D, antacids and steroids; uric acid stones with salicylate and probenecid; and crystalline stones from triamterene, indinivir and aciclovir.

Stones can only form in urine that is supersaturated with the chemical constituents of that stone. Urinary inhibitors of calcification and stone formation (e.g. increased urinary citrate or a more alkaline urine pH) are also important. Clinical manifestations are typically loin (often radiating to groin) pain (ureteric colic) and visible haematuria. The pain comes in waves and can be excruciatingly severe, causing vomiting.

The basic evaluation of a patient with a renal stone is shown in Box 6.2.

Box 6.2 **Basic evaluation of renal stone formers**

- Stone history: how many stones, age at first onset, one or both kidneys, need for intervention
- Medical history
- Medications

- Family history
- Physical examination
- Laboratory tests
  - urine: microscopy and culture
  - pH
  - stone chemical analysis
  - urea and electrolytes, chloride, bicarbonate, uric acid, calcium, phosphate
  - PTH, if calcium elevated
- Radiological investigations
  - KUB
  - CT IVU
  - ultrasound

General treatment of renal stones involves relief of pain (preferably using parenteral non-steroidal anti-inflammatory drugs or opiates), exclusion of urinary obstruction and eradication of infection. Acute surgical intervention may be needed. Prevention of future stone formation or symptomatic episodes is important and is summarized in Box 6.3.

Box 6.3 **Prevention of future/recurrent stone formation**

- Increase in fluid intake (to > 3 L/day)
- Limit salt intake (which decreases urinary calcium excretion)
- Increase oral calcium intake (binding dietary oxalate)
- Decrease urinary calcium excretion (thiazide diuretic)
- Reduce dietary oxalate (for oxalate stone formers)

Renal cysts and tumours

In modern hospitals and institutions there is much more ready access to, and use of, renal/abdominal ultrasound and CT scanning. As a result, there are more renal cysts and masses incidentally discovered than before (Figure 6.3). The key question is the assessment of the risk of malignancy. Ultrasound imaging is only 80%

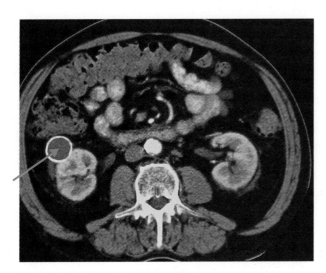

Figure 6.3 Single large calcified renal cyst.

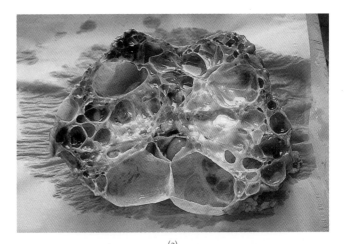

(a)

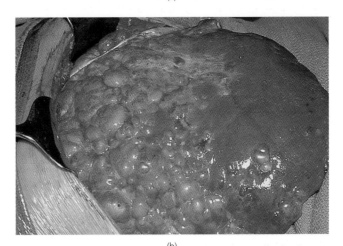

(b)

Figure 6.4 Polycystic kidney disease: (a) kidney and (b) cysts in liver.

sensitive at detecting renal parenchymal lesions; CT and MRI scanning are much more sensitive techniques. Figure 6.4 shows polycystic kidney disease.

Any solid mass with a diameter > 3 cm should be regarded as potentially malignant and be removed, unless circumstances prevent this. Proximity of a solid renal mass to the renal vein may well determine tumour behaviour as much as the mass's absolute diameter. Mixed solid–cystic lesions present significant difficulties. Causes of renal cystic disease are given in Box 6.4.

Box 6.4 **Renal cystic diseases**

Non-genetic

- Simple cysts (increasingly common in those aged > 50 years)
- Medullary sponge kidney
- Medullary cystic disease
- Acquired multicystic disease (in advanced CKD).

Genetic

- Autosomal dominant polycystic disease (mostly adults)
- Von Hippel Lindau disease

- Tubero-sclerosis
- Autosomal recessive polycystic disease (mostly children)
- Nephronophthisis
- Multicystic/dysplastic syndromes

Autosomal dominant polycystic kidney disease

Autosomal dominant polycystic kidney disease (ADPKD), an important cause of hypertension and renal failure in adults, may rarely present in infancy and childhood:

- antenatal ultrasound: discrete cysts in fetal kidneys (although in some people the cysts do not appear until their teens);
- visible haematuria;
- hypertension, renal failure;
- incidental finding of renal cysts during abdominal ultrasound.

ADPKD has no gender or race preference. There may not be a known family history of this condition, and, occasionally, the affected parent is only diagnosed by ultrasound performed after the condition is detected in their child. See also Figure 6.4b (cysts are seen in the liver in 50% of patients).

ADPKD can cause cysts in the liver and problems in other organs, such as the heart and blood vessels in the brain. In the United States, about 500 000 people have ADPKD, and it is the fourth-leading cause of kidney failure.

ADPKD is one of the most common inherited disorders. The phrase 'autosomal dominant' means that if one parent has the disease there is a 50% chance that the disease will pass to a child. Either the mother or father can pass it on, but new mutations may account for a quarter of new cases.

Many people with ADPKD live for decades without developing symptoms. For this reason, ADPKD is often called 'adult polycystic kidney disease'.

Symptoms of ADPKD

The most common symptoms are pain in the back and the sides (between the ribs and hips), and headaches. The dull pain can be temporary or persistent, mild or severe.

People with ADPKD can also experience:

- UTIs
- haematuria
- liver and pancreatic cysts
- abnormal heart valves
- high blood pressure (BP)
- kidney stones
- cerebral and other aneurysms
- diverticulosis.

Diagnosis of ADPKD

To diagnose ADPKD, the ultrasound should show three or more kidney cysts. Typically, there are many more than this and the cysts often distort the shape of the kidney as well as cause it to enlarge.

The diagnosis is strengthened by a family history of ADPKD, and the presence of cysts in other organs.

Once the condition is established in one family member, it is good practice to offer to screen other family members too. In the case of children (< 15 years old), a normal ultrasound scan cannot guarantee that there is no ADPKD and so it is not recommended to screen children until they have reached early adulthood: the cysts can develop and become manifest only in adult life. It is very unusual, however, for a normal screening ultrasound to be falsely negative (or normal) with a subject aged > 20 years.

A genetic test can detect mutations in the PKD1 and PKD2 genes. Although this test can detect the presence of the ADPKD mutations before cysts develop, its usefulness is limited by two factors: it cannot predict the onset or ultimate severity of the disease, and no absolute cure is available to prevent the onset of the disease. On the other hand, a young person who knows of an ADPKD gene mutation may be able to forestall the disease through diet and BP control. The test may also be used to determine whether a young member of an ADPKD family can safely donate a kidney to a parent. Anyone considering genetic testing should receive counselling to understand all the implications of the test.

Treatment of ADPKD

Although a cure for ADPKD is not yet available, treatment can ease the symptoms and may help to prolong life. Novel approaches and therapies may soon be clinically available.

Renal, back and cyst pain

These can be caused by kidney stones, UTIs, cyst infection or cyst haemorrhage. Therapies include bed rest and antibiotics and, much more rarely, cyst aspiration under ultrasound or CT guidance. High BP is very common indeed in ADPKD, though keeping BP under control, unfortunately, has little effect on the progression of ADPKD.

Pregnancy in chronic kidney disease

Pregnancy may be the first time that young women have their BP checked, or urine tests performed, so a small number of pregnant women are discovered to have haematuria, proteinuria, pyuria, raised BP or renal impairment.

Non-visible haematuria can be detected in up to 25% of normal pregnancies at some stage. This disappears in the majority after delivery. Causes include glomerular disease, pre-eclampsia and UTI. Visible haematuria (formerly known as macroscopic haematuria;) is rare, and most often due to urine infection.

The development of significant proteinuria during pregnancy always requires evaluation and investigation. Up to 95% of pregnant women excrete less than 200 mg protein/24 h. A protein:creatinine ratio > 30 mg protein/mmol creatinine is abnormal (i.e. the upper limit of normal for PCR is 30 in pregnancy compared to 15 in the non-pregnant state). Persistent *de novo* proteinuria in pregnancy is most often due to pre-eclampsia, when raised BP is typically seen in the second half of pregnancy. Significant proteinuria in pre-eclampsia confers a higher risk of adverse maternal and fetal outcome. Proteinuria due to pre-eclampsia should resolve within a few months of delivery, so persistent proteinuria suggests that pregnancy has unmasked prior renal disease.

There is no specific treatment for proteinuria in pregnancy; ACEI and ARB are contra-indicated because of unwanted fetal side-effects. If the pregnant woman becomes nephrotic, there is a direct relationship between maternal plasma albumin and birth weight. Renal biopsy can safely be performed in pregnancy, and depending on the result, specific treatment, including immuno-suppression, can be considered.

Asymptomatic bacteriuria affects 2–10% of all women and can lead to serious complications in pregnancy (acute pyelonephritis and sometimes premature delivery) so is worth screening for (urine dipstick/nitrites, then culture if positive) and treating (amoxicillin/clavulanic acid, nitrofurantoin or second-generation cephalo-sporin). It is more common in women with urological, anatomical or functional abnormalities, diabetic women, and older multiparous women. The overall incidence of pyelonephritis in pregnancy is approximately 1% (usually second trimester), but amongst women with asymptomatic bacteriuria it can be as high as 25%.

Acute kidney injury (AKI) in pregnancy was a feature of around 1 in 2000 pregnancies in the 1960s; the commonest reasons being septic abortion, or in the third trimester obstetric haemorrhage or eclampsia. AKI requiring dialysis in the modern era is much rarer; causes include antepartum haemorrhage, pre-eclampsia, urinary obstruction, sepsis and haemolytic-uraemic syndrome. Rapid restoration of circulating volume (if depleted) is vital for maternal and fetal outcome.

Fertility rapidly declines with advancing CKD, so few women with significant reduction of renal function become pregnant; there is an increased rate of fetal loss, and early delivery is more common in established CKD. Renal function can worsen irreversibly with pregnancy. Pregnancy while on dialysis is very unusual indeed, and delivery of a live infant is truly exceptional. Significant proteinuria, and starting pregnancy with abnormal renal function, are bad prognostic (fetal and maternal renal function) features. Renal transplantation, if successful, can restore fertility and the chance of successful delivery; prednisolone, azathioprine, ciclosporin and tacrolimus are safe drugs to take in pregnancy (though breast feeding is often not recommended because of entry of these drugs into breast milk). Other newer immunosuppressants require more extensive research before we can be certain of their safety profiles. Mycophenolate mofetil, for example, is now known to be terato-genic. It should be avoided in women hoping to conceive and replaced by azathioprine (when appropriate so to do).

Further reading

Bisceglia M, Galliani CA, Senger C, Stallone C, Sessa A (2006) Renal cystic diseases: A review. *Adv Anat Pathol* **13**(1): 26–56.

Stratta P, Canavese C, Quaglia M (2006) Pregnancy in patients with kidney disease. *J Nephrol* **19**(2): 135–43.

Sutters M (2006) The pathogenesis of autosomal dominant polycystic kidney disease. *Nephron Exp Nephrol* **103**(4): 149–55.

Taylor EN, Curhan GC (2006) Diet and fluid prescription in stone disease. *Kidney Int* **70**(5): 835–9.

CHAPTER 7

Adult Nephrotic Syndrome

Richard Hull[1], Sean Gallagher[1] and David Goldsmith[2]

[1]Guy's and St Thomas' NHS Foundation Trust, London, UK
[2]King's College London, London, UK

OVERVIEW

- Nephrotic syndrome (NS) is a common condition in kidney specialist practice with significant complications. It is caused by a wide range of primary (idiopathic) and secondary glomerular diseases.

- Patients can present in various clinical settings, with not insignificant numbers undergoing community-based treatment with care shared between specialists and primary care.

- All patients need referral to a nephrologist for further investigation with a renal biopsy.

- Initial management should be focused at investigating its cause, identifying complications and managing the presenting symptoms of the disease.

- No conclusive evidence currently exists for the best treatment strategies for most primary glomerular diseases.

Box 7.1a Diagnostic criteria for nephrotic syndrome

- Greater than 3–3.5 g/24 hr proteinuria or spot urine PCR of > 300–350 mg/mmol
- Serum albumin < 25 g/L
- Clinical evidence of peripheral oedema
- Can also be associated with hyperlipidaemia (raised total cholesterol) and lipiduria

---

Box 7.1b Definition and classification of proteinuria (see Chapter 1)

- Transient increased proteinuria can be seen in fever, post-exercise, post-seizure, in severe acute illnesses
- Persistent proteinuria of > 150 mg/day (PCR ~ 10–20 mg/mmol) implies renal or systemic disease
- Dipsticks predominantly detect urinary albumin (and are positive if excretion is > 300 mg/day)

Nephrotic syndrome

The nephrotic syndrome (NS) is one of the best-known presentations of adult or paediatric kidney disease (Orth and Ritz 1998). It describes the association of heavy *proteinuria* with *peripheral oedema, hypoalbuminaemia* and *hyperlipidaemia* (Box 7.1a, b). NS has multiple causes, significant complications and requires referral to a nephrologist for further investigation and management. Patients can present *de novo* in various clinical settings, with not insignificant numbers of patients undergoing community-based treatment, with management shared between specialists and primary care (the paradigm for much of renal medicine in the twenty-first century).

Though NS is a common condition in nephrological practice and should feature in the differential diagnosis of any oedematous patient, there can be uncertainty about how best to manage it. In part this is due to a lack of randomized controlled trials, and the presence of only a handful of Cochrane systematic reviews.

This chapter provides an update on the management of NS in adults. We review relevant investigation and therapeutic strategies

for the general condition of NS, and for some of the primary glomerular causes (but we deliberately avoid highly specialized or recherché conditions). In particular, our approach emphasizes the clinical challenges faced by doctors without specialized renal experience when presented with a patient with suspected NS.

When considering renal oedema, salt and water retention and the action of diuretics, it is helpful to have in mind an understanding of both renal anatomy and physiology at the level described in Figure 7.1.

Conditions causing nephrotic syndrome

NS is caused by a wide range of conditions that can be classified as primary (idiopathic) glomerular (Table 7.1) or secondary diseases (Box 7.2).

Primary (idiopathic) glomerular disease

Primary glomerular diseases account for the majority of cases of NS. Thirty years ago, idiopathic membranous nephropathy (see Appendix 2) was the most common primary cause. The incidence

---

ABC of Kidney Disease, Second edition.
Edited by David Goldsmith, Satish Jayawardene and Penny Ackland.

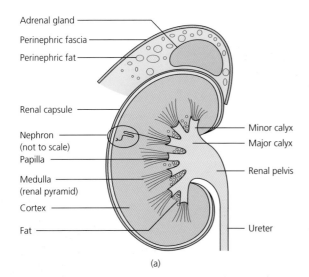

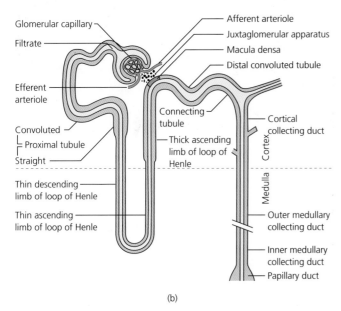

Figure 7.1 (a) Kidney structure. (b) Nephron anatomy. (*Source:* Adapted from *The Renal System at a Glance*, with permission of Blackwell Publishing Ltd.)

of the other glomerular pathologies, particularly focal segmental glomerulosclerosis (FSGS) (see Appendix 2), has increased. There are marked racial associations with different underlying primary glomerular diseases: membranous nephropathy is the most frequent

Table 7.1 Primary glomerular diseases causing the nephrotic syndrome.

Disease	Frequency of disease (%)		
	Classic data		Modern data
	< 60 yr	> 60 yr	
Focal segmental glomerulosclerosis	15	2	35
Membranous	40	39	33
Minimal change	20	20	15
Membranoproliferative, e.g. IgA	7	0	14
Other diseases	18	39	3

(*Source:* Data adapted from Haas *et al.* 1997 and Orth and Ritz 1998.)

Box 7.2 Secondary causes of nephrotic syndrome

- Diabetes mellitus
- Neoplasia
- Drugs
  - gold
  - antimicrobials
  - NSAIDs
  - penicillamine
  - captopril
  - tamoxifen
  - lithium
- Infections
  - HIV
  - hepatitis B and C
  - mycoplasma
  - syphilis
  - malaria
  - schistosomiasis
  - filariasis
  - toxoplasmosis
- SLE
- Amyloid
- Miscellaneous

cause of NS in Caucasians, while FSGS is the cause of 50–57% of cases of NS in black patients. (Haas *et al.* 1997; Korbet *et al.* 1996).

Secondary glomerular disease

A wide range of diseases and drugs can cause NS. Secondary causes can often give a similar or identical histological lesion to a primary disease but have an identifiable underlying pathological process. Diabetic nephropathy is, and will remain, the commonest cause. Amyloid is also an important cause of NS; in one series AL amyloid nephropathy accounted for 10% of cases (Haas *et al.* 1997).

The pathophysiological reasons for nephrotic syndrome

The size-selective and charge-selective filtration barrier of the glomerulus prevents the passage of proteins across it. There are three layers: the fenestrated endothelium, the glomerular basement membrane and podocytes with the slit diaphragm between their foot processes (Figures 7.2 and 7.3). NS develops from protein leakage caused by injuries to this barrier. These alter its charge and size selectivity through effects on podocytes by immune and non-immune mechanisms, and to the expression of vital adhesion molecules such as nephrin.

Explanations for oedema in nephrotic syndrome

The underlying process behind sodium retention and oedema formation is complex, controversial and not fully resolved.

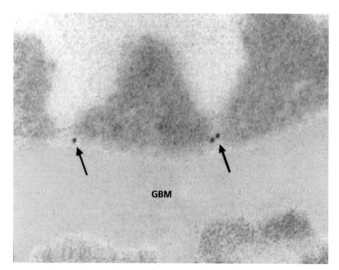

Figure 7.2 Glomerular slit diaphragm. (*Source:* Reproduced with permission from Institute of Biotechnology, Helsinki.)

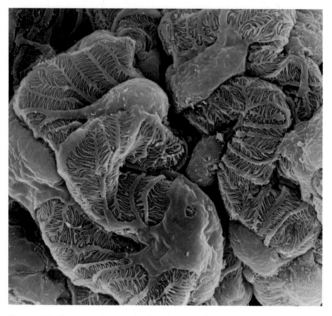

Figure 7.3 Electron micrograph of podocyte cells. (*Source:* Reproduced with permission from Steve Gschmeissner/Science Photo Library.)

The classic 'underfill' hypothesis proposes that low plasma oncotic pressure resulting from proteinuria and hypoalbuminaemia leads to intravascular volume depletion. The physiological response, via the renin-angiotensin-aldosterone and sympathetic nervous systems, causes sodium retention and thus oedema. There are many clinical and experimental studies that tried to validate this theory; a detailed exposition is beyond the scope of this review (Deschênes *et al.* 2003; Koomans 2003). The alternative 'overfill' theory proposes that the processes causing sodium retention are intrarenal, primarily in the collecting duct of the nephron (Ichikawa *et al.* 1983). There are still unanswered questions and, indeed, one rather more pragmatic view is that sodium retention leading to oedema formation (Figure 7.4) is likely to result from a spectrum of pathogenic mechanisms; some 'underfill' and some 'overfill' (Hamm and Batuman, 2003).

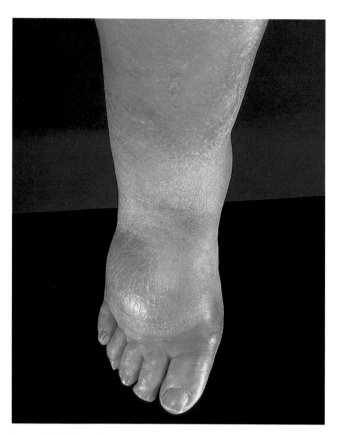

Figure 7.4 Pitting oedema.

Complications of nephrotic syndrome

NS has systemic consequences (Box 7.3). Not infrequently, the first manifestation of NS can be a complication, such as deep venous thrombosis (DVT), breathlessness or infection. There is overproduction of proteins in the liver (as part of the hepatic response to hypoalbuminaemia) and loss of low molecular weight proteins in the urine. Significant changes in the protein environment of the body result in many of the complications seen. It is important for the clinician to be aware of their potential and actively prevent their occurrence.

Box 7.3 **Complications of nephrotic syndrome**

- Thromboembolism
  - ○ DVT +/− pulmonary embolism
  - ○ renal vein
  - ○ arterial (rare)
- Infection
  - ○ cellulitis
  - ○ bacterial peritonitis (rare)
  - ○ bacterial infections, e.g. pneumonia
  - ○ viral infections in the immunocompromised
- Hyperlipidaemia
- Malnutrition
- Acute kidney injury

Risk of thromboembolism

NS results in a hypercoagulable state with an increased risk of thromboembolic events. Embolism affect up to 10% of adults in clinical series of NS (Nolasco *et al.* 1986). Multiple abnormalities in the coagulation system occur, including increased plasma levels of pro-coagulant factors, reduced plasma levels of anticoagulant factors, abnormal platelet function, altered endothelial function and decreased fibrinolytic activity. Intravascular volume depletion, an increase in haematocrit from diuretics, and immobilization are significant contributory factors.

The most common sites of thrombosis in adults are the deep veins of the lower limb. This is often asymptomatic. Renal vein thrombosis (RVT) is a well-recognized, though uncommon, complication of NS and is said to be more common when NS is caused by membranous nephropathy or amyloidosis. Pulmonary embolism is also a potential consequence. Arterial thrombosis, affecting mesenteric, axillary, femoral, ophthalmic, renal, pulmonary and coronary arteries has also been (much more rarely) reported.

Infection

Infection can occur in up to 20% of adult patients with NS and is a significant cause of morbidity and, occasionally, mortality. Patients have an increased susceptibility to infection from low serum IgG concentrations, reduced complement activity and depression of T cell function (Ogi *et al.* 1994).

A variety of infectious complications, particularly bacterial, can occur. Cellulitis is common, especially in severely oedematous limbs, due to skin splits or punctures. Spontaneous bacterial peritonitis is a serious but rare infection in adults. It can present insidiously with mild abdominal colicky pain or as fulminant sepsis. *Streptococcus pneumoniae* and gram-negative organisms are the most frequent causative bacteria. Viral infections have been linked to relapses in minimal change NS. Infections are a risk in patients receiving immunosuppressive treatment for NS.

Acute kidney injury

This is a rare complication of NS. It can happen as a consequence of excessive diuresis, interstitial nephritis related to diuretic or nonsteroidal anti-inflammatory drug (NSAID) use, sepsis and RVT. It can happen spontaneously, usually at presentation and occurs more often in older patients. Patients can require dialysis and can take weeks to months to recover (Crew *et al.* 2004).

Assessing the patient presenting with nephrotic syndrome

The key aims are to assess the current clinical state of the patient, ensuring no complications are present, and to begin to formulate whether there is a primary or secondary cause underlying the syndrome. The vast majority of patients will require referral to a nephrologist for further management, including (in adults) a renal biopsy. Patients can present with complications of the syndrome with the actual diagnosis being made later (e.g. DVT).

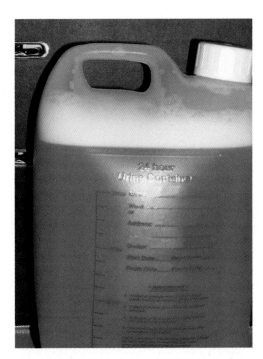

Figure 7.5 Frothy urine.

History

A thorough and careful history is important in elucidating the cause of NS. Patients can notice breathlessness, leg and facial swelling and, more rarely, frothy urine (protein acting like a detergent in the urine [Figure 7.5]). Particular note should be made of any features suggestive of systemic disease, for example systemic lupus erythematosus (SLE), drug history (especially any recent or new medications, be they prescribed or over the counter) as well as any acute or chronic infections. It is important to remember the links with malignancy particularly of the lungs and large bowel. A history of chronic inflammation may point towards a diagnosis of secondary amyloid. A family history is also important, as there are a number of congenital causes of NS.

Clinical signs

Patients usually present with increasing peripheral oedema (Figure 7.4). Up to four litres of fluid can remain clinically undetectable. Oedema is often first noticed peri-orbitally and it can become very severe with lower leg and genital oedema as well as ascites, pleural and pericardial effusions. It is important to mention to the non-specialist that neither raised blood pressure (BP) nor elevated jugular venous pressure/pulmonary oedema are cardinal features of NS. If these are present, it is more likely that one is dealing with (acute) nephritic syndrome (e.g. secondary to acute glomerulonephritis) or there is significant cardiac or renal failure. The BP in NS can be low, normal or raised: this depends on many factors, including previous history of raised BP, underlying cause of NS, renal function, extracellular fluid volume status and cardiac function.

Features of the underlying disorder may be evident, such as the butterfly facial rash of SLE or the neuropathy and retinopathy associated with diabetes mellitus.

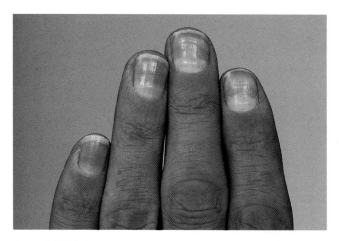

Figure 7.6 Nail changes.

Hyperlipidaemia is one of the classic accompaniments to the condition and eruptive xanthomas can appear. The nails can show white bands due to persistent hypoalbuminaemia (Figure 7.6).

Investigations

Initial investigations (Box 7.4) help establish the current clinical status and pin down the underlying cause of the NS. Key steps

---

Box 7.4 **Investigations in the nephrotic patient**

Haematology

- full blood count
- coagulation screen
- ESR

Chemistry

- urea and electrolytes including eGFR
- LFT including albumin
- bone profile
- lipid profile
- glucose
- CRP
- spot urine for protein:creatinine ratio (preferably early morning)

Microbiology

- Hepatitis B and C and HIV serology (after appropriate consenting)
- MSU
- blood cultures if there is fever (> 38°C)

Immunology

- antinuclear antibody (ANA)
- anti-double-stranded DNA antibody (dsDNA)
- complement levels (C3 and C4)
- serum immunoglobulins and electrophoresis
- urine for Bence Jones Protein

Radiology

- renal ultrasound
- CXR
- other imaging (dependent on clinical signs and suspicion of malignancy)

---

include assessment of the renal function through measurement of serum urea and creatinine and an estimated glomerular filtration rate (eGFR). The urine should be assessed for the presence of haematuria (suggesting glomerulonephritis) and proteinuria (3 plus protein indicates nephrotic range). It is important to measure the amount of protein being excreted. A spot urine sample for a protein:creatinine ratio (PCR) is almost as accurate, less prone to error and gives quicker results than a 24-hour urine collection (Gaspari *et al.* 2006). Nephrotic-range proteinuria is defined as a PCR greater than 300–350 mg/mmol. A renal ultrasound, giving an assessment of renal size and morphology, should be performed early, and should be done urgently if there is suspicion of RVT.

General treatment measures for nephrotic syndrome

Oedema

The underlying cause of the oedema is sodium retention. The aim of therapy is to create a negative sodium balance. Dietary sodium limitation (< 100 mmol/day), fluid restriction and diuretics may all be needed. Oedema should be reversed by engineering a steady diuresis to cause a weight loss of around 0.5–1 kg/day (and so daily weight is an important metric). More zealous diuresis can precipitate acute kidney injury from volume depletion, electrolyte disturbances (hyponatraemia, hypokalaemia) and thrombo-embolism due to haemoconcentration.

Loop diuretics such as furosemide or bumetamide are commonly used. Starting doses should be in the 'conventional' range (e.g. 40–80 mg of furosemide orally). Oedema of the gut wall can affect the absorption of diuretics; refractory cases respond best to larger doses of intravenous loop diuretics. Intravenous boluses or preferably infusions (of much higher doses) of loop diuretics are commonly used; there can be severe side-effects from large (intravenous) doses of loop diuretics (e.g. electrolyte derangement, deafness or photo-sensitive skin blistering), so care must be taken.

To try to improve on poor responses found with loop diuretics, thiazide diuretics or potassium-sparing diuretics are often added to treatment regimens. A typical additional agent is metolazone (2.5–5 mg daily). These agents inhibit downstream sodium reabsorption and thus work in synergy with loop diuretics which induce a more proximal natriuresis (Figure 7.7). This loop diuretic–thiazide combination can be tremendously effective, and so requires careful oversight usually in hospital, with daily weight, BP and electrolyte monitoring.

Although intravenous (salt-poor) albumin infusion has often been used to improve or initiate diuresis (working, it is surmised, by increasing the delivery of the diuretic to its site of action through increasing the amount of plasma-bound drug, and by expanding plasma volume), this practice is not supported by evidence from studies. There are potential harmful consequences flowing from the use of intravenous albumin, such as anaphylaxis, hypertension and pulmonary oedema (Mees 1996).

Proteinuria

Whereas a healthy individual will normally excrete less than 150 mg protein (or 20–30 mg albumin) per day in the urine daily,

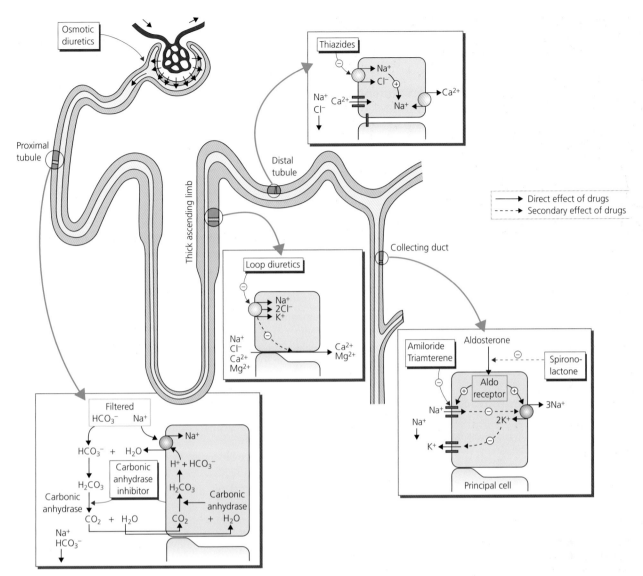

Figure 7.7 Site of action of diuretics in the kidney. (*Source:* Adapted from *The Renal System at a Glance*, with permission from Blackwell Publishing Ltd.)

nephrotic syndrome is associated with greater than 3000–3500 mg/24 h of proteinuria. One of the main goals of treatment is the reduction or elimination of proteinuria. Proteinuria is the best independent predictor of progression in all renal disease (Ruggenenti *et al.* 1998). Strategies to limit protein excretion will also serve to help correct oedema. In some patients this can be achieved by treating the underlying pathology, but in the majority of patients the proteinuria needs active control. The general measures used usually achieve proteinuria reduction by also causing a reduction in glomerular filtration rate (GFR). A number of older treatments, for example high-dose NSAIDs, have significant side-effects and are rarely used now. Low protein diets have not shown consistent results in reducing proteinuria, and are not recommended.

Proteinuria is linked to BP – for heavily nephrotic patients a BP of < 125/75 mmHg is ideal. Proteinuria is also linked to obesity, so weight loss in chronically heavily proteinuric obese subjects is desirable.

Angiotensin converting enzyme inhibitors (ACEI), either on their own or in conjunction with angiotensin II receptor antagonists, are the mainstay of anti-BP/antiproteinuric therapy. The dose response curve in this setting is different from their antihypertensive effects (which can mean using larger doses) and it can often take some weeks for their full effect to be manifest. Proteinuria reduction can be seen in the absence of any effect on systemic BP; combination therapy reduces proteinuria more effectively than single agents alone (Nakao *et al.* 2003; Tsouli *et al.* 2006). Using these agents mandates regular monitoring of plasma electrolytes (also mandatory when large diuretic doses are employed). (See Chapters 1 and 3).

It should not be forgotten that indapamide, and non-dihydropyridine calcium-channel blockers such as verapamil and diltiazem, are all ant-proteinuric antihypertensives, and these can also usefully be added to ACEI-based regimens.

In extreme cases, where the proteinuria is severe and uncontrollable leading to incapacitating symptoms from, or complications of, NS (e.g. renal dysfunction or malnutrition), it is possible to use nephrectomy or renal arterial embolization. In practice, these extreme measures are very rarely needed in adults.

Thromboembolism: prevention and treatment

Any confirmed thrombosis needs systemic anticoagulation with heparin and then warfarin. Higher doses than normal of heparin may be needed as its site of action, antithrombin III, can be greatly reduced in NS. There are no reliable indicators of the risk of thromboembolism to guide prophylaxis. General factors need to be addressed such as immobility from severe oedema, treatment of sepsis and avoidance of haemoconcentration by excessive diuretic use. Because there is no strong evidence base, there are difficulties in deciding to whom to give prophylactic anticoagulation, and for how long. The factors above (immobility, oedema and haemoconcentration) need to be taken into account, as should the presence of any other pro-coagulant state, but there is no definite threshold of proteinuria or hypoalbuminaemia to signify risk of complications. It is common practice to anticoagulate with heparin and warfarin for as long as the serum albumin is less than 20 g/L with nephrotic-range proteinuria. There will be situations, for example pregnancy, where heparin (typically low molecular weight) alone is used.

Use of prophylactic antibiotics

There are conflicting views on the use of antibiotic and vaccine prophylaxis. There are no trials assessing the use of prophylactic antibiotics in adults. A Cochrane review in 2004 could not recommend any interventions for preventing infections in NS (Wu *et al.* 2004).

Treatment of NS-associated dyslipidaemia

Hyperlipidaemia is a common feature of NS. Numerous abnormalities in lipids occur, including increases in hepatic production of apolipoprotein (apo) B-containing lipoproteins, such as very-low-density lipoproteins (VLDL), low-density lipoproteins (LDL) and lipoprotein(a), as well as alterations in high-density lipoprotein (HDL) levels and impaired removal of cholesterol from the periphery.

There is evidence of increased cardiovascular events in nephrotic patients that could be related to the lipid abnormalities (Ordonez *et al.* 1993), but as yet no prospective trials show treatment improves survival. There is some evidence from meta-analysis and post-hoc analysis that controlling cholesterol levels improves glomerular function and prevents progression of renal disease in chronic kidney disease (CKD), especially those with proteinuria (Sandhu *et al.* 2006). Thus, it is advisable to treat persistent hyperlipidaemia as one would in the general population. Treating the underlying cause of NS and thereby reducing proteinuria will improve or resolve the dyslipidaemia.

Dietary changes used in NS patients

Muscle wasting is a major problem in severe NS and patients have a greatly increased albumin turnover. The optimal protein intake for such patients is not clear. A low protein diet runs risks of negative nitrogen balance, and arguments can be made for normal or high protein diets.

Salt and water retention are the cause of the oedema in NS. For these reasons, it is prudent to salt-restrict NS patients to < 100 mmol sodium per day. Careful judgement of diuretic dose, fluid intake and dietary salt restriction is needed.

Management of primary and secondary glomerular diseases causing nephrotic syndrome

The primary glomerular diseases that can cause NS have differing significances for the patient with NS, both in terms of treatment strategy and renal prognosis (a detailed discussion is beyond the scope of this chapter; interested readers are directed to the reference texts in the Further resources section below).

Minimal change nephropathy causing NS has been treated with immunosuppressive agents, primarily corticosteroids, since the 1950s. Over the years, many other agents such as cyclophosphamide, mycophenolate, and calcineurin inhibitors (ciclosporin and tacrolimus) have been used to try to improve responses in steroid-insensitive, frequently relapsing or poorly responding cases. More recherché therapies are beyond the scope of this chapter. There is still no consensus on the treatment of the different causes of the NS or any definitive answers from randomized controlled trials. Awareness of the use of immunosuppressive agents is very important, as many have significant side-effects (Box 7.5).

Minimal change nephropathy has an excellent prognosis with many patients maintaining their renal function in the long term. The majority of patients respond to a course of corticosteroids; many, however, can relapse and remain steroid-dependent, sometimes requiring additional agents for achievement of remission.

FSGS patients always have nephrotic or non-nephrotic proteinuria. Patients with secondary FSGS have a hyperfiltration injury and should be treated with ACE inhibitors or angiotensin II receptor antagonists. Most untreated patients with primary FSGS will develop CKD stage 5 from 5 to 20 years after presentation with response to therapy remaining the best prognostic indicator of outcome. Patients often need long courses of high-dose prednisolone, and additional agents, to achieve some remission. Patients who do show remission have a better long-term renal outcome than those who do not.

Membranous nephropathy is an immune mediated glomerular disease associated with malignancy in 7–15% patients aged over 60 years old. It has a variable renal prognosis. Up to 30% of patients remit spontaneously, while 30% progress to CKD stage 5 within 5–15 years. The best treatment strategy remains controversial, especially in view of the high spontaneous remission rates. A Cochrane meta-analysis in 2004 concluded that there was no long-term effect of immunosuppressive treatment on patient and/or renal survival (Schieppati *et al.* 2004). Most nephrologists feel a trial of immunosuppressive therapy is warranted in patients with idiopathic membranous nephropathy who remain nephrotic despite maximal use of ACE inhibitors and angiotensin receptor blockers (ARBs), and in those who have deteriorating renal function.

It is not possible to review all of the evidence for intervention in secondary glomerular pathology leading to NS, but it is noteworthy

---

Box 7.5 **Major side-effects of commonly used immunosuppressive agents for nephrotic syndrome**

Immunosuppressive agents all increase the susceptibility to and severity of infection.

Corticosteroids (e.g. prednisolone)

- gastrointestinal effects
  - gastritis
  - ulceration
- proximal myopathy
- osteoporosis
- Cushingoid changes
- hypertension
- glucose intolerance

Cyclophosphamide

- bone marrow depression
- infection
- alopecia
- sterility and effects on reproductive function
- haemorrhagic cystitis
- bladder carcinoma
- nausea and vomiting

Ciclosporin

- renal impairment (long term)
- hepatic dysfunction
- tremor
- hyperkalaemia
- hypertension
- hyperlipidaemia
- gingival hypertrophy

Tacrolimus

- diabetes mellitus
- hyperkalaemia
- hypertension
- gastrointestinal disturbances
- hepatic dysfunction
- renal impairment

Mycophenolate mofetil

- leucopoenia
- GI disturbance especially diarrhoea and vomiting

Other agents

- Levamisole
  - gastrointestinal effects

---

that, for example, successful intervention to resolve amyloid fibril formation (in both immunocyte- and inflammation-associated amyloidosis) can lead to complete resolution of all proteinuria.

Conclusions

NS is a common condition in nephrological practice and can present in diverse ways in different healthcare settings. It has significant complications. Though one can standardize the investigation and the general management, long-term control of NS remains incomplete, as currently we are unable effectively to combat several primary glomerular diseases that can cause NS. Large randomized trials to ascertain the best management of the primary glomerular pathologies responsible for much of NS are overdue.

References

Crew RJ, Radhakrishnan J, Appel G (2004) Complications of the nephrotic syndrome and their treatment. *Clin Nephro* **62**: 245–59.

Deschênes G, Feraille E, Doucet A (2003) Mechanisms of oedema in nephrotic syndrome: old theories and new ideas. *Nephrol Dial Transplant* **18**: 454–56.

Gaspari F, Perico N, Remuzzi G (2006) Timed urine collections are not needed to measure urine protein excretion in clinical practice. *Am J Kidney Dis* **47**(1): 1–7.

Haas M, Meehan SM, Karrison TG, Spargo BH (1997) Changing etiologies of unexplained adult nephrotic syndrome: a comparison of renal biopsy findings from 1976–1979 and 1995–1997. *Am J Kidney Dis* **30**: 621–31.

Hamm LL, Batuman V (2003) Edema in the nephrotic syndrome: new aspects of an old enigma. *J Am Soc Nephrol* **14**: 3008–16.

Ichikawa I, Rennke HG, Hoyer JR *et al.* (1983) Role for intrarenal mechanisms in the impaired salt excretion of experimental nephrotic syndrome. *J Clin Invest* **71**: 91103.

Koomans HA (2003) Pathophysiology of oedema in idiopathic nephrotic syndrome. *Nephrol Dial Transplant* **18**(suppl 6): vi30–vi32.

Korbet SM, Genchi RM, Borok RZ, Schwartz MM (1996) The racial prevalence of glomerular lesions in nephrotic adults. *Am J Kidney Dis* **27**: 647–51.

Mees, EJD (1996) Does it make sense to administer albumin to the patient with nephrotic oedema ? *Nephrol Dial Transplant* **11**: 1224–6.

Nakao N, Yoshimura A, Morita H *et al.* (2003) Combination treatment of angiotensin-II receptor blocker and angiotensin-converting-enzyme inhibitor in non-diabetic renal disease (COOPERATE): a randomised controlled trial. *Lancet* **361**: 117–24.

Nolasco F, Cameron JS, Heywood EF *et al.* (1986) Adult-onset minimal change nephrotic syndrome: a long-term follow-up. *Kid Int* **29**: 1215–23.

Ogi M, Yokoyama H, Tomosugi N *et al.* (1994) Risk factors for infection and immunoglobulin replacement therapy in adult nephrotic syndrome. *Am J Kidney Dis* **24**: 427–36.

Ordonez JD, Hiatt RA, Killebrew EJ, Fireman BH (1993) The increased risk of coronary heart disease associated with nephrotic syndrome. *Kid Int* **44**: 638–42.

Orth SR, Ritz E (1998) The nephrotic syndrome. *N Engl J Med* **338**: 1202–11.

Ruggenenti P, Perusa A, Mosconi L, Pisone R, Remuzzi G (1998) Urinary protein excretion is the best predictor of ERF in non-diabetic chronic nephropathies. *Kid Int* **53**: 1209–16.

Sandhu S, Wiebe N, Fried LF, Tonelli M (2006) Statins for improving renal outcomes: a meta-analysis. *J Am Soc Nephrol* **17**(7): 2006–16.

Schieppati A, Perna A, Zamora J *et al.* (2004) Immunosuppressive treatment for idiopathic membranous nephropathy in adults with nephrotic syndrome. *Cochrane Database of Systematic Reviews* **18**: CD004293.

Tsouli SG, Liberopoulos EN, Kiortsis DN, Mikhailidis DP, Elisaf MS (2006) Combined treatment with angiotensin-converting enzyme inhibitors and angiotensin II receptor blockers: a review of the current evidence. *J Cardiovasc Pharmacol Ther* **11**: 1–15.

Wu HM, Tang JL, Sha ZH, Cao L, Li YP (2004) Interventions for preventing infection in nephrotic syndrome. *Cochrane Database Syst Rev* **2**: CD003964.

Further resources

For doctors

Burden R, Tomson C (2005) Identification, management, and referral of adults with chronic kidney disease: concise guidelines. *Clinical Medicine*; **5**: 635–42. Available online at URL http://www.renal.org/eGFR/eguide .html.

Davison AM, Cameron JS, Grünfeld J-P *et al.* (eds) (2005) *Oxford Textbook of Clinical Nephrology*, 3rd edn. Oxford University Press, Oxford.

http://bestpractice.bmj.com/best-practice/monograph/356.html (2011) version due out any day now).

Orth SR, Ritz E (1998) The nephrotic syndrome. *N Engl J Med* **338**: 1202–11.

Steddon SJ, Ashman N, Cunningham J, Chesser A (eds) (2006) *Oxford Handbook of Nephrology and Hypertension.* Oxford University Press, Oxford.

For patients

The National Kidney Federation UK (http://www.kidney.org.uk). The federation of UK kidney patient groups has a collection of disease resources under the 'Medical information' heading.

The Renal Unit of the Royal Infirmary of Edinburgh, Scotland, UK (http://renux.dmed.ed.ac.uk/edren/index.html) is an excellent source of information about renal disease for patients and non-specialist practitioners.

CHAPTER 8

Renal Artery Stenosis

Philip Kalra[1], Satish Jayawardene[2] and David Goldsmith[3]

[1]Hope Hospital, Salford, UK
[2]King's College Hospital NHS Foundation Trust, London, UK
[3]King's College London, London, UK

OVERVIEW

- Renal artery stenosis (RAS) may present as drug-resistant hypertension, acute kidney injury (especially with angiotensin converting enzyme inhibitor (ACEI) or angiotensin receptor blocker (ARB) use), chronic renal impairment or recurrent flash pulmonary oedema.

- The most common pointers to clinical diagnosis of RAS are the presence of femoral, renal or aortic bruits and the coexistence of severe extra-renal vascular disease.

- RAS should be considered when marked deterioration in renal function (e.g. $\geq$30% increase in creatinine or $\geq$ 25% fall in eGFR) occurs when an ACEI or ARB is used.

- Atheromatous renovascular disease (ARVD) is the cause of 90% of cases of RAS, and it can be unilateral or bilateral.

- Post-mortem studies indicate the presence of ARVD in over 40% of older patients. ARVD does not cause significant hypertension or chronic kidney disease (CKD) in the majority of patients.

- Approximately 5–10% of RAS cases are due to fibromuscular dysplasia (FMD), typically found in hypertensive young women. Angioplasty can cure hypertension in about a third of this group of patients.

- There are several screening methods for RAS.

- Both renal arteriography and angioplasty have significant risks to the patient, which should be considered.

- Renal artery angioplasty and stenting are effective at improving renal artery stenoses for both ARVD and FMD. However, only in FMD can one expect a significant improvement in blood pressure (BP) control in the majority of patients.

- ARVD should be considered as part of a diffuse vascular disease process, and management should involve control of hypertension and hyperlipidaemia, use of antiplatelet agents and cessation of smoking.

- ACEI and ARBs are amongst the optimal anti-hypertensive choices for patients with ARVD, although care and specialist advice may be necessary if marked renal deterioration is found following the administration of such medication.

Definition and background

Renal artery stenosis (RAS) is a reduction in the lumen of one or both renal arteries, and can be an important cause of renal failure and secondary hypertension. In >90% of cases the condition is due to atheroma of the renal arteries (atheromatous renovascular disease, or ARVD; Figure 8.1), and this is a disease of ageing. Patients usually have evidence of atheroma in other important vascular beds, such as coronary artery disease (CAD), cerebrovascular and peripheral vascular disease (PVD), and RAS involves the renal ostia (renal arterial origins) in 90% of cases. ARVD can be unilateral or bilateral and up to 50% of patients have renal artery occlusion (RAO) at diagnosis. It is very common: post-mortem studies indicate its presence in over 40% of older patients.

Approximately 5–10% of RAS cases are due to fibromuscular dysplasia (FMD; Figure 8.2), which, when it is discovered, is

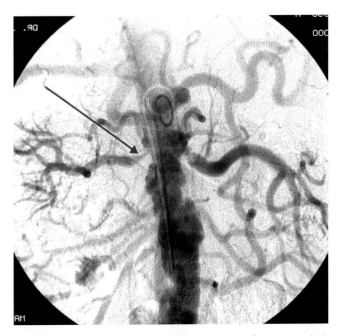

Figure 8.1 Renal arteriogram showing atheromatous renal artery stenosis. A flush aortogram: note the irregular shape of the aorta due to atheroma. The red arrow points to marked reduction in the arterial lumen of the renal artery. Atheromatous RAS typically involves the ostia of the renal arteries, as these are involved with aortic atherosclerotic lesions.

ABC of Kidney Disease, Second edition.
Edited by David Goldsmith, Satish Jayawardene and Penny Ackland.
© 2013 John Wiley & Sons, Ltd. Published 2013 by John Wiley & Sons, Ltd.

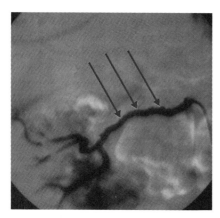

Figure 8.2 Renal arteriogram showing fibromuscular renal artery stenosis. A selective right renal artery angiogram in fibromuscular RAS (FMD). The aorta is not affected by atheroma. The red arrows point to multiple bead-like irregularities in the lumen of the renal artery well away from the ostium. A nephrogram can be seen, and there is contrast in the renal collecting system and ureter.

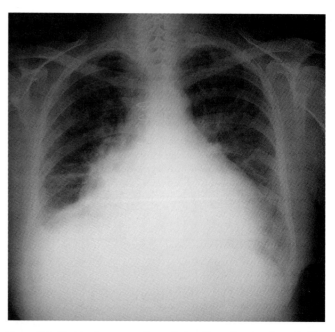

Figure 8.3 'Flash' pulmonary oedema. A chest X-ray showing shows florid bilateral pulmonary oedema, which was the presentation of severe RAS in this patient.

typically seen in hypertensive young women, most of whom have well-preserved renal function. In contrast to ARVD, angioplasty of FMD RAS lesions is usually associated with clinical improvement, such as cure of hypertension in a third of patients.

Although many patients with ARVD will have hypertension and/or chronic kidney disease (CKD), in the vast majority of patients it is likely to be incidental and pathophysiologically insignificant to these latter conditions. This explains the inconsistent results following renal artery intervention in ARVD, which has led to uncertainty in guidelines for its management. Assessing the severity of a stenosis and having a thorough understanding of the clinical context are essential to planning management. Most RAS will be suspected, diagnosed and treated in a hospital setting. One important exception is a change in renal function with the introduction of angiotensin converting enzyme inhibitors (ACEIs) or angiotensin receptor blockers (ARBs), as numerically the majority of scripts for hypertension and heart failure are community-based.

Clinical features

Although the majority of ARVD cases are asymptomatic, the condition should be suspected in patients presenting with renal dysfunction and hypertension who have evidence of atheromatous disease in other vascular beds. Particular clinical features include significant deterioration of renal function (e.g. $\geq 30\%$ increase in serum creatinine or $\geq 25\%$ fall in estimated glomerular filtration rate, or eGFR) accompanying use of ACEI or ARBs, or unexplained 'flash' (sudden onset) pulmonary oedema (Figure 8.3), but the presence of femoral, renal or aortic bruits and the coexistence of severe extra-renal vascular disease are the commonest clinical pointers to diagnosis. Hypertension may be absent, particularly in patients with chronic cardiac dysfunction, but a high index of suspicion for RAS diagnosis is advised in cases with severe (often systolic) hypertension, especially when unresponsive to three or more anti-hypertensive agents and with evidence of widespread

vascular disease. Box 8.1 lists some of the important clinical clues to the presence of RAS.

Box 8.1 **Clinical clues to the presence of renal artery stenosis**

- Onset of hypertension < 40 years of age
- Drug-resistant hypertension
- Chronic renal impairment in an atherosclerotic patient
- Recurrent flash pulmonary oedema
- Widespread arterial disease
- Vascular bruits (particularly epigastric and/or renal)
- Asymmetrical renal size (> 10% difference) on renal ultrasound
- Development of significant renal impairment with the introduction of an ACEI/ARB (30% or more increased creatinine or >25% decreased eGFR)

Pathogenesis of renal dysfunction in patients with renal artery stenosis

Most interventional treatments for RAS are undertaken with the aim of controlling severe hypertension or reversing, or at least stabilizing, renal dysfunction. In the case of FMD, such treatment is usually justified: here, the hypertension and renal impairment are often consequent upon renal ischaemia due to 'hydraulic' effects of the renal arterial narrowing. As the patient is typically young and the kidney beyond the RAS has not been subjected to years of hypertensive and atherosclerotic injury, revascularization can be expected to improve these clinical abnormalities.

However, this is not generally the case with ARVD. There is now compelling evidence that intra-renal injury, probably most often due to long-standing hypertension, dyslipidaemia and inflammation (all of which pre-date RAS development), is the major factor responsible for renal dysfunction in the majority of patients who have CKD with ARVD. Hence, there is often little correlation between severity of RAS and the extent of renal dysfunction in ARVD, and patients with unilateral RAS can develop renal failure even though the contralateral renal artery remains patent. Proteinuria appears to be a key marker of this intra-renal injury and it is strongly linked to baseline renal function as well as long-term outcome. The histological changes of 'ischaemic nephropathy' include a constellation of hypertensive damage, cholesterol athero-embolism, intra-renal vascular disease and sclerosing glomerular lesions. These associations help explain the variable outcomes that occur following renal revascularization procedures, which are discussed later.

Investigations

Screening and diagnostic investigations generally assess relative renal size and renal arterial anatomy, but additional tests (e.g. isotope GFR, which can be used to measure function of individual kidneys) are needed to correlate function with these morphologic parameters. Captopril renography is now rarely used, except perhaps in patients with both severe hypertension and preserved renal function.

Asymmetric renal size (>1.5 cm difference in bipolar length) at ultrasound is suggestive, but there are many other explanations for such inequality and ARVD is often bilateral. Doppler ultrasonography can be a sensitive screening test but it is time-consuming, highly operator-dependent (and hence not a cost-effective screening tool) and thus few centres presently offer this facility. Contrast-enhanced CT angiography has an excellent detection rate but, as with conventional intra-arterial angiography (which used to be termed the 'gold standard' investigation for RAS), there is a risk of contrast nephrotoxicity in higher-risk patients (e.g. those with GFR <30 mL/min, diabetics). In high-risk patients radiocontrast procedures should be limited where possible, and alternative imaging should be considered. Intravascular volume depletion is a key risk factor, which can be corrected by appropriate volume expansion with intravenous saline. Oral use of the antioxidant *N*-acetylcysteine has been widely assessed with conflicting results and its role remains uncertain. However, it is an inexpensive agent without significant side-effects and its use in clinical practice may not therefore be inappropriate.

Contrast-enhanced MR angiography (MRA) is becoming the favoured imaging method for the proximal renal vasculature (Figure 8.4). It is sensitive, and gadolinium is non-nephrotoxic at low doses; patient suitability is limited by claustrophobia or by the presence of metallic objects (e.g. aneurysm clips). Recent concerns about fibrosing skin problems seen in patients with advanced CKD and exposure to gadolinium – nephrogenic systemic fibrosis or nephrogenic fibrosing dermopathy (NSF/NFD) – need fuller evaluation. Noteworthy advances in MR techniques include the possibility of measuring individual renal function, with the potential of providing a comprehensive functional and anatomical scan in a single visit.

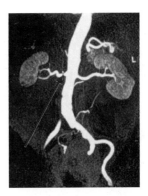

Figure 8.4 Magnetic resonance angiogram showing renal artery stenosis. An MRA with intravenous gadolinium contrast enhancement showing aortic irregularity and a tight right renal artery stenosis indicated by the arrow – distally, a smaller kidney compared to the other side.

Management of renal artery stenosis

In those patients where RAS is an incidental finding with little or no hypertension, no invasive intervention is generally required. As stated previously, renal revascularization, usually with angioplasty alone, is likely to be successful in controlling or even curing hypertension, and in reversing renal dysfunction (when it occurs) in FMD (Box 8.2).

Box 8.2 **The management of renal artery stenosis**

- Maximal BP control (may require more than six different antihypertensive drugs)
- Renal artery angioplasty plus stenting for flash pulmonary oedema, severe drug-resistant hypertension, and for preservation of renal function
- Statin to reduce hypercholesterolaemia, especially in atherosclerotic RAS
- Low-dose aspirin therapy

Medical treatment

ARVD should be considered as part of a diffuse vascular disease process rather than as a solitary disease affecting the renal circulation. Extra-renal vascular comorbidities should not be overlooked, as they may be the major contributor to the poor outcome of ARVD patients. An evidence base to guide best medical 'vascular protective' management is lacking, but attention to limiting the progression of atheromatous disease by control of hypertension and hyperlipidaemia, use of antiplatelet agents and cessation of smoking seem non-controversial approaches. Although it may appear counterintuitive, both ACEI and ARBs would be optimal anti-hypertensive choices for patients with ARVD, especially for those with proteinuric chronic parenchymal disease, and those with coexisting CAD and cardiac dysfunction. However, this could only be responsibly undertaken with very careful supervision. In these situations there needs to be a balance between, for example, renal risk and benefit, versus cardiac and cerebral protection. Needless to say, to date no randomized controlled trial has addressed this difficult question.

Renal revascularization

Revascularization procedures have been utilized for the treatment of RAS for over three decades, but percutaneous interventional techniques – angioplasty with/without stent placement (Figures 8.5 and 8.6) – has now largely replaced surgical revascularization, accounting for 95% of all procedures in ARVD. Nevertheless, these procedures should only be performed after careful patient evaluation as complications can occur. Some degree of contrast nephropathy and cholesterol embolization occurs in a large proportion of patients, but they are clinically significant in only a minority; renal arterial rupture or thrombosis are fortunately uncommon. Until now, only four randomized clinical trials have investigated the outcome after revascularization in ARVD – none showed any benefit to renal function (but the trials were small and were not adequately powered to do so), but most showed a modest improvement in hypertension control after angioplasty. There are numerous retrospective reports from individual centres, and these have rarely taken the revascularization technique into consideration: only a minority of the patients (<25%) showed an improvement in renal function. The overall effect upon renal functional outcome in the whole ARVD group is generally minimal. Large-scale randomized clinical trials are essential to determine the overall effects of intervention, and to help identify which subgroups of patients will benefit from revascularization. The ASTRAL trial reported in 2009 that there was no identifiable medical benefit (blood pressure, BP, control or GFR preservation) for the performance of renal arterial angioplasty or stenting.

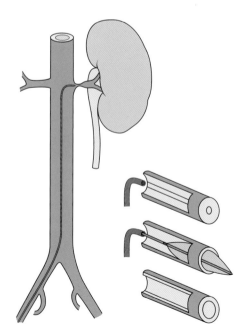

Figure 8.5 Cartoon of renal artery angioplasty.

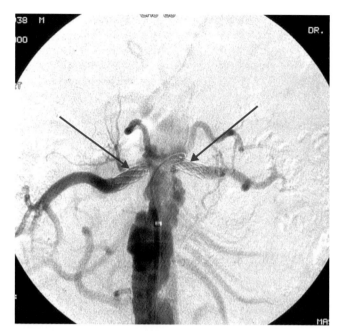

Figure 8.6 Bilateral renal artery stents. A flush aortogram shows the presence of bilateral proximal renal artery stents (the red arrows point to these at the ostia of the renal arteries, just protruding into the aortic lumen).

Despite the remaining uncertainties over the place of renal revascularization in the majority of patients with ARVD, few would dispute its necessity in patients presenting with recurrent 'flash' pulmonary oedema in association with a high-grade RAS lesion, as the procedure can be life-saving. There is also reasonable consensus that revascularization should be considered in patients with high-grade RAS and the following clinical scenarios:

- severe hypertension resistant to all medical therapy;
- when a patient who requires ACEI or ARB therapy (e.g. for cardiac failure) presents with significant ACEI-related renal dysfunction;
- when there is evidence of recent-onset RAO in a reasonably sized kidney. Such patients present with anuria (if the RAO affects someone with a solitary kidney) and rapidly deteriorating renal function. Angioplasty (possibly with prior thrombolytic therapy) can dramatically rescue the functioning renal mass in this situation.

Prognosis of patients with atheromatous renovascular disease

Only a minority of patients with CKD and ARVD progress through to need dialysis, the remainder usually dying from cardiovascular complications; a recent US epidemiological study showed that the risk of death of ARVD patients during follow-up was almost six times that of developing end stage renal failure (ESRF). The poor survival relates to patient age but is largely due to the effects of comorbid cardiovascular disease. In studies from Hope Hospital, ARVD patients have been shown to have a five-year survival of 52%, but those presenting with ESRF had a 30-fold relative risk of mortality compared with patients with well-preserved function; patients with CAD had significantly higher mortality than patients with isolated ARVD.

Further reading

ASTRAL Investigators, Wheatley K, Ives N *et al.* (2009) Revascularization versus medical therapy for renal-artery stenosis. *N Engl J Med* **361**(20): 1953–62.

Hegarty J, Wright JR, Kalra PR, Kalra PA (2006) The heart in renovascular disease: An association demanding further investigation. *Int J Cardiol* **111**(3): 339–42.

Krumme B, Donauer J (2006) Atherosclerotic renal artery stenosis and reconstruction. *Kidney Int* **70**(9): 1543–7.

Textor SC (2006) Renovascular hypertension update. *Curr Hypertens Rep* **8**(6): 521–7.

CHAPTER 9

Palliative Care for Patients with Chronic Kidney Disease

Frances Coldstream[1], Neil S. Sheerin[2] and Emma Murphy[1]

[1]Guy's and St Thomas' NHS Foundation Trust, London, UK
[2]Newcastle University and Medical School, Newcastle, UK

OVERVIEW

- Patients need to be given timely information about prognosis and quality of life, whether they are on dialysis, choose to stop or even choose not to start dialysis in the first place.

- Patients with stages 4–5 chronic kidney disease (CKD) often have slowly progressive disease and may survive many months or even years without dialysis. However, prediction of survival can be difficult and patients can deteriorate rapidly, have a slow steady decline in function or a decline punctuated by recurrent acute problems.

- In some patients dialysis may offer little or no significant survival rate improvement.

- There is increased recognition of a need for coordinated management of end-of-life care for patients with end stage renal failure (ESRF).

- For patients who choose not to dialyse, it is important to offer treatment for other aspects of CKD, e.g. erythropoietin therapy and phosphate control.

- Symptoms such as pain, dry skin, itching, nausea and vomiting, constipation, anorexia, muscle cramps, abdominal bloating, insomnia and fatigue all need to be considered and treated where possible.

- Collaboration with palliative care services may be appropriate.

Introduction

As with any major organ failure, severe renal disease (stage 5 chronic kidney disease (CKD) or estimated glomerular filtration rate (eGFR), or glomerular filtration rate (GFR) <15 mL/min) is associated with significant morbidity and increased mortality. Over the last three decades, long-term renal replacement with dialysis has become increasingly available to older people and those with greater comorbidity. However, it is now recognized that continuing or initiating dialysis may not always offer an improved quantity or quality of life; indeed, we run the risk of worsening patient outcome. In this context, palliative (also referred to as conservative,

supportive or end-of-life) treatment options should be part of our management of renal failure. We need to offer realistic choices to patients with end stage renal failure (ESRF) but can only do so if appropriate services and support are in place.

Which renal patients need palliative care?

Palliative care is important for many patients with ESRF. For the majority, if not all patients, end-of-life issues should be addressed prior to the introduction of renal replacement therapy. Dialysis is, after all, a treatment and not a cure. Recognizing the need for palliative care in patients with ESRF is challenging. This is largely due to unpredictable illness trajectories often influenced by comorbidities. Murray *et al.* (2005) suggest we ask the question, 'would I be surprised if my patient were to die in the next 12 months?' If the answer is no, the clinician should be considering if such a person has palliative care needs. Recent evidence has shown the question to be a more accurate predictor of prognosis than previously proposed variables, such as plasma albumin. In the United Kingdom, a general practice initiative called the Gold Standards framework can help both identify patients and then improve their care. This approach could apply to patients who are deteriorating despite dialysis, those who choose not to have dialysis or those who would not tolerate dialysis and are treated conservatively. Patients may also choose or be advised to stop dialysis, perhaps because of the development of intercurrent illness, which may make dialysis medically impossible, or there may be an acknowledgement of a failure to tolerate, or benefit from, dialysis treatment.

The extent of the clinical need

The number of patients requiring dialysis has increased steadily, and is predicted to continue to rise for the next 20 years. Older people receiving haemodialysis will constitute a major proportion of this increase due to the high incidence of renal failure in this group (Figure 9.1) and the increasing age of the population (Figure 9.2). The incidence of dialysis-requiring renal failure increases with age, peaking at 567 per million population (pmp) in males over 80 years of age. This compares with 45 pmp in men in their 20s. This may underestimate the true incidence of ESRF due to unrecognized or unreferred renal failure.

ABC of Kidney Disease, Second edition.
Edited by David Goldsmith, Satish Jayawardene and Penny Ackland.
© 2013 John Wiley & Sons, Ltd. Published 2013 by John Wiley & Sons, Ltd.

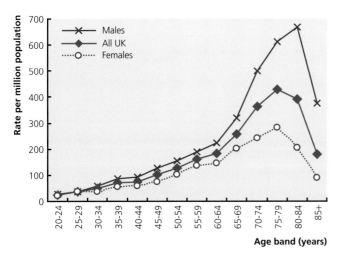

Figure 9.1 Renal replacement therapy (RRT) incidence rates by age and gender in 2009. The overall peak is in the 75–79 age band. (*Source*: Cawskey *et al.* (2010) UK Renal Registry. See References.)

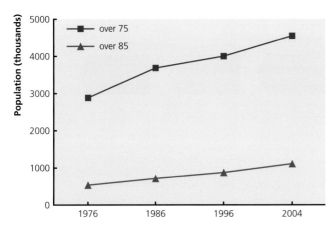

Figure 9.2 Chronic kidney disease stages 4–5. (*Source:* Data from the National Statistics Office.)

The older group of patients has a high level of comorbidity. Around 67% of patients over the age of 65 commencing dialysis have one or more significant comorbidities that may adversely affect survival. Age and comorbidity are strongly linked in dialysis candidates; comorbidity is one factor that contributes to high mortality rates on dialysis, with 28% of patients over 85 years old dying in the first 90 days of starting dialysis, and this in selected patients for whom it was thought dialysis would be beneficial.

This need for coordinated management of end-of-life care for patients with ESRF has been recognized in the National Service Framework for Renal Services (Box 9.1). This has both acknowledged this important phase of patient care and set a series of standards for the delivery of end-of-life care to patients with renal disease (Box 9.2). In addition, the UK CKD guidelines recommend referral or discussion of all people who have stage 4 or 5 CKD to nephrology services for an assessment, even if it is thought that dialysis will not be appropriate (e.g. terminal malignancy, terminal cardiac or lung disease). More recently, the *End of Life Care strategy* (Department of Health 2008) stated that palliative care should be provided on the basis of need not diagnosis, followed by *End of*

life care in advanced kidney disease: A framework for implementation (NHS Kidney Care 2009) which aimed to raise the quality of end-of-life care for kidney patients (Figure 9.3). These government guidelines have been important in the development of renal palliative services, recognizing the clinical need and incorporating emerging evidence.

Box 9.1 Need for coordinated management of end-of-life care

'People with end stage renal failure receive timely evaluation of their prognosis, information about the choices available to them, and for those near end-of-life a jointly agreed palliative care plan, built around their individual needs and preferences.'
Source: Department of Health (2005).

Box 9.2 Standards for the delivery of end-of-life care

The renal multi-skilled team has access to expertise in the discussion of end-of-life issues, including those of culturally diverse groups and varied age groups, the principles of shared decision making, training in symptom relief relevant to advanced non-dialysed end stage renal failure (ESRF).

Prognostic assessment based on available data offered to all patients with stage 4 CKD as part of the preparation for RRT (renal replacement therapy).

People receive timely information about the choices available to them, such as ending RRT and commencing non-dialytic therapy, and have a jointly agreed palliative care plan built around individual needs and preferences.

People who are treated without dialysis receive continuing medical care including all appropriate non-dialytic aspects of CKD, and wherever possible are involved in decisions about medication options.

Individuals are supported to die with dignity, and their wishes met wherever practicable regarding where to die, their religious and cultural beliefs, and the presence of the people closest to them.

The care plan includes culturally appropriate bereavement support for family, partners, carers and staff.
Source: Department of Health (2005).

Conservative management of patients choosing not to dialyse

Conservative management is now a recognized treatment modality in nephrology, with more than 20–25% of the United Kingdom's predialysis population selecting this option. The decision not to dialyse can only be made after discussion between the multidisciplinary renal team and the patient, relatives and carers. The patient needs to be given information about prognosis and quality of life with or without dialysis (Figure 9.4). Information about this is scarce. Although emerging evidence demonstrates the survival advantage of dialysis in patients aged >75 years, it is substantially reduced by comorbidity and ischaemic heart disease in particular.

Patients with stages 4–5 CKD often have slowly progressive disease and may survive many months or even years without dialysis. If patients are assessed appropriately, it is possible to identify those

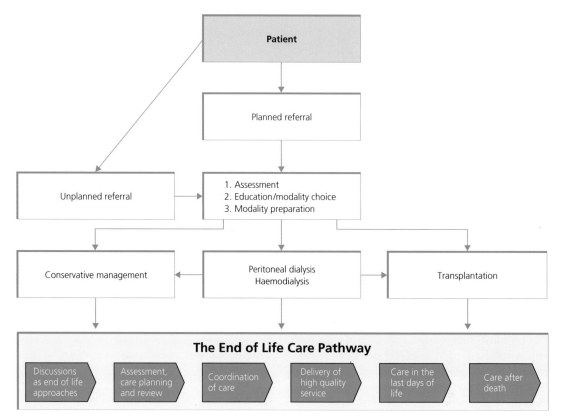

Figure 9.3 The pathway for the management of advanced kidney disease recognizes the importance of an end of life care pathway for all ESRF patients regardless of treatment modality. (*Source:* NHS 2009.)

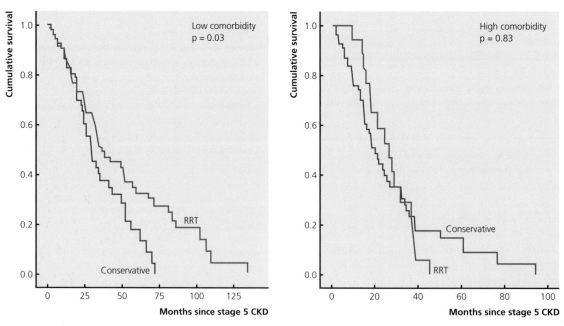

Figure 9.4 Comparison of Kaplan-Meier survival curves by modality (RRT vs conservative kidney management) in patients >75 years. The panel on the left depicts the relationships in those with low comorbidity and that on the right in those with high comorbidity.

for whom dialysis offers little or no significant survival advantage and advise accordingly. However, predicting survival, with or without dialysis, can be difficult. Patients can deteriorate rapidly, have a slow steady decline in function or a decline punctuated by recurrent acute problems. A study carried out by Murtagh and colleagues

(2011) reported for the first time a distinctive renal trajectory contrasting with that previously described in other conditions. Patients managed conservatively (without dialysis) have a steep functional decline in the late stages of their disease. This has important implications for delivery of care; renal and palliative services need to be rapidly responsive to changing needs in this population as function declines in the last months and weeks of life.

It is important that this is not seen as a 'no treatment' option, and patients are offered treatment for other aspects of CKD, for example erythropoietin therapy and phosphate control. We also need to be able to actively support these patients as end of life approaches. For some patients choosing dialysis, there may be few easy treatment options. Unit-based haemodialysis will typically require patients to travel to a unit, which may be geographically distant, three times per week for dialysis treatment. The effect of treatment and its complications (e.g. infection related to dialysis access) on quality of life, particularly in older patients with significant comorbidity, can be great and needs to be considered thoroughly when planning management.

Withdrawal from dialysis

Patients may actively choose to withdraw from dialysis, or dialysis may be stopped if it is no longer providing clinical benefit. In the United Kingdom, withdrawal from dialysis is now the commonest cause of death after the first 90 days in patients aged over 75 years.

The prognosis after withdrawal of dialysis depends on coexisting illness and residual renal function. Residual renal function is progressively lost on dialysis, particularly haemodialysis, and many dialysis patients may eventually become anuric. In the presence of severe illness, death will usually occur within three days. Studies have consistently reported the mean survival after dialysis withdrawal to be 8–10 days with a range of 1–46 days. Key issues to consider before stopping dialysis include:

- the exclusion of reversible factors;
- anticipation of symptoms (as pre-existing symptoms prior to dialysis withdrawal may intensify as death approaches);
- additional comorbid illness, residual renal function and duration of dialysis therapy can aid prognostication.

Symptoms: identification and control

The symptom burden related to ESRF is perhaps greater than previously thought, even in those patients on renal replacement therapy (Box 9.3). Studies of symptom prevalence suggest that symptoms may be as frequent and as severe in ESRF as in malignant disease or other progressive chronic diseases (Table 9.1). This is true not only in patients withdrawing from or not dialysing but also in patients actively dialysing. Symptoms such as anorexia, anxiety and depression are common to many chronic, progressive diseases, while others such as pruritus and restless legs may be more specific to renal disease. Control of symptoms can prove difficult with the added complexity of altered drug excretion in ESRF. Recent studies have indicated the likely efficacy of the World Health Organization (WHO) analgesic ladder to manage pain in ESRF patients (see Appendix 1).

Anaemia, so common in CKD stages 4 and 5, can easily be treated with iron and, where needed, erythropoietin therapy (see Chapter 5). Breathlessness can be ameliorated by managing anaemia, by giving oxygen, by treatment of acidosis with oral sodium bicarbonate and by treatment of fluid overload with diuretics.

Table 9.1 Comparison of symptoms in end stage renal failure on dialysis with other end-of-life populations.

Symptom prevalence (%)	ESRF (%)	Cancer (%)	Chronic obstructive pulmonary disease (%)	Heart disease (%)
Pain	47–50	35–96	34–77	41–77
Depression	5–60	3–77	37–71	9–36
Fatigue	73–87	32–90	68–80	69–82
Sleep disorder	31–71	9–69	55–65	36–48
Breathlessness	11–62	10–70	90–95	60–88
Anorexia	25–62	30–92	35–67	21–41
Nausea	30–43	6–68	–	17–48

Source: Data from a systematic review of the literature by Solano *et al.* (2006) shows the minimum and maximum reported incidence of each symptom.

Clonazepam can be useful in restlessness, while gabapentin can help uraemic pruritus and neuropathy (but needs to be used sparingly as it can accumulate). Pain relief can be effected by trans-cutaneous patches, for example fentanyl and buprenorphine, rather than primary use of oral opiates, which accumulate significantly in renal failure.

> **Box 9.3 Symptom burden related to end stage renal failure**
>
> - Fatigue and lack of energy
> - Itching
> - Pain
> - Sleep disturbance
> - Restless legs
> - Anxiety and/or depression
> - Anorexia
> - Constipation
> - Cough and dyspnoea
> - Nausea and vomiting

Unless specifically asked, patients will often under-report symptoms. A systematic approach, perhaps based on symptom questionnaires, may therefore be useful. Patients with ESRF may also have symptoms due to comorbid conditions that may require specific intervention. Formal symptom assessment tools validated in ESRF patients include:

- The renal version of the Patient Outcome Scale: symptom module (POSs renal);
- The Dialysis Symptom Index (DSI), developed from the Memorial Symptom Assessment Scale by Weisboard;
- The modified Edmonton Symptom Assessment Scale (ESAS).

Advanced planning

With patients who choose not to dialyse or for patients who express a wish to withdraw from dialysis, early advance planning is key. This should include discussing what treatment a patient would want during an acute deterioration in health, describing what resuscitation means and whether an intensive therapy unit (ITU) admission should take place. In addition, discussion about preferred place of care (including preferred place of death) should be included. Some patients may want to formalize their wishes by writing them down. It is likely that advanced directives will be increasingly used in this context. The healthcare team need to accurately document and communicate the patient's wishes to all individuals involved in the patient's care. It is essential to ensure that these decisions and plans are regularly revisited to ensure they are still in line with the wishes of the patient and that the appropriate care options are in place.

Links with palliative care services

Palliative care for non-cancer diseases is a rapidly developing area. As with other organ failure, there are both generic and disease-specific considerations for the treatment of patients with ESRF. There needs to be close collaboration between existing renal and palliative services, both community- and hospital-based, to develop management pathways for ESRF patients.

Conclusions

Patients will start under the care of renal services and as their disease progresses and their end of life approaches they will need increasing palliative input. This change needs to be as seamless as possible. It may include a long period during which both services are involved in the care of an individual patient, as well as an extended multidisciplinary group including general practitioners, nursing services, occupational and physiotherapists, counsellors and chaplains (Box 9.4).

Box 9.4 **End-of-life issues**

- Symptom management
- Social support
- Psychological support
- Spiritual care
- Carer support
- Bereavement support

References

Caskey F, Dawnay A, Farrington K, Feest T, Fogarty D, Inward C, Tomson CRV (2010) Nephron Clinical Practice Vol. 119, Suppl. 2, 2011. UK Renal Registry 2010 13th Annual Report of the Renal Association. UK Renal Registry, Bristol, UK. *Notice: The data reported here have been supplied by the UK Renal Registry of the Renal Association. The interpretation and reporting of these data are the responsibility of the authors and in no way should be seen as an official policy or interpretation of the UK Renal Registry or the Renal Association.*

Chandna SM, Da Silva-Gane M, Marshall C et al. (2011) Survival of elderly patients with stage 5 CKD: comparison of conservative management and renal replacement therapy. *Nephrol Dial Transplant* 26(5): 1608–14.

Department of Health (2008) End of Life Care Strategy: promoting high quality care for all adults at end of life, http://www.dh.gov.uk/prod_consum_dh /groups/dh_digitalassets/@dh/@en/documents/digitalasset/dh_086345 .pdf.

Murray SA, Boyd K, Sheikh A (2005) Palliative care in chronic illness. *BMJ* 330(7492): 611–12.

Murtagh FEM, Sheerin N, Addington-Hall J, Higginson IJ (2011) Trajectories of illness in stage 5 chronic kidney disease: A longitudinal study of patients' symptoms and concerns in the last year of life. *Clin J Am Soc Nephrol* 6: 1580–1590.

NHS (2009) *End of Life Care in Advanced Kidney Disease: A framework for implementation.* London: National Health Service, http://www.endoflife careforadults.nhs.uk/publications/eolcadvancedkidneydisease.

Solano JP, Gomes B, Higginson IJ (2006) A comparison of symptom prevalence in far advanced cancer, AIDS, heart disease, chronic obstructive pulmonary disease and renal disease. *J Pain Symptom Manage* 31(1): 58–69.

Further reading

Addington-Hall JM, Higginson IJ (eds) (2001) *Palliative Care Needs for Non-Cancer Patients.* Oxford University Press, Oxford.

Barakzoy AS, Moss AH (2006) Efficacy of the World Health Organization analgesic ladder to treat pain in end-stage renal disease. *J Am Soc Nephrol* 17: 3198–3203.

Chambers EJ, Germain M, Brown E (eds) (2004) *Supportive Care for the Renal Patient.* Oxford University Press, Oxford.

Cohen LM, Germain M, Poppel DM et al. (2000) Dialysis discontinuation and palliative care. *Am J Kidney Dis* 36(1): 140–144.

Davison SN, Jhangri GS, Johnson JA (2006) Cross-sectional validity of a modified Edmonton Symptom Assessment System in dialysis patients: A simple assessment of symptom burden. *Kidney Int* 69: 1621–5.

Davison SN (2005) Chronic pain in end-stage renal disease. *Ad Chron Kid Dis* 12(3): 326–34.

Department of Health (2005) *National Service Framework for Renal Services: Part 2: Chronic Kidney Disease, Acute Renal Failure, and End of Life Care.* HMSO, London.

Holley JL (2005) Palliative care in end-stage renal disease: Focus on advance care planning, hospice referral, and bereavement. *Semin Dialysis* 18(2): 154–6.

Launay-Vacher V, Karie S, Fau JB et al. (2005) Treatment of pain in patients with renal insufficiency: The World Health Organization three-step ladder adapted. *J Pain* 6: 137–48.

Murphy EL, Murtagh FE, Carey I, Sheerin NS (2009) Understanding symptoms in patients with advanced chronic kidney disease managed without dialysis: Use of a short patient-completed assessment tool. *Nephron Clin Pract* 111: c74–c80.

Murtagh F, Chai MO, Donohoe P et al. (2007) The use of opioid analgesia in end-stage renal disease patients managed without dialysis: Recommendations for practice. *J Pain Palliat Care Pharmacother* 21: 5–17.

Murtagh FE, Marsh JE, Donohoe P et al. (2007) Dialysis or not? A comparative survival study of patients over 75 years with chronic kidney disease stage 5. *Nephrol Dial Transplant* 22: 1955–62.

Murtagh FEM, Murphy E, Sheerin N (2008) Illness trajectories: An important concept in the management of kidney failure. *Nephrol Dialy Transplant* 23: 3746–8.

Smith C, Da Silva-Gane M, Chandna S et al. (2003) Choosing not to dialyse: Evaluation of planned non-dialytic management in a cohort of patients with end-stage renal failure. *Nephron Clinical Practice* 95(2): c40–c46.

Weisbord SD, Fried LF, Arnold RM et al. (2004) Development of a symptom assessment instrument for chronic hemodialysis patients: The Dialysis Symptom Index. *J Pain Symptom Manage* 27: 226–40.

CHAPTER 10

Dialysis

Christopher W. McIntyre[1] and James O. Burton[2]

[1]Department of Renal Medicine, Derby City Hospital, Derby, UK
[2]Department of Infection, Immunity & Inflammation, School of Medicine and Biological Sciences, University of Leicester, Leicester, UK

OVERVIEW

- Indications to commence dialysis are:
  - intractable hyperkalaemia;
  - acidosis;
  - uraemic symptoms (nausea, pruritus, malaise);
  - therapy-resistant fluid overload;
  - chronic kidney disease (CKD) stage 5.
- There is considerable variation of the level of glomerular filtration rate (GFR) individuals may tolerate before becoming markedly uraemic.
- 'Crash-landing' onto dialysis confers a reduction in patient survival that persists for at least the first three years of subsequent therapy.
- Early identification and assiduous preparation mentally and physically are needed in the predialysis phase for those likely to need renal replacement therapy (RRT).
- Haemodialysis (HD) involves circulating blood through a disposable dialyser. The vascular access of choice is the arteriovenous fistula (AVF). This, however, requires suitable peripheral veins and needs four to eight weeks for the fistula to mature. If there are no suitable veins, a graft can usually be inserted. Acute access with venous catheters has a high complication rate.
- Peritoneal dialysis (PD) involves using the peritoneum as the dialysis membrane, with pre-packaged fluid being instilled into the peritoneal space via a Tenckhoff catheter. This is usually only inserted once the decision to start dialysis is made.
- HD is usually performed in four-hour sessions, three times a week, in hospital-based dialysis units.
- PD typically involves continuous ambulatory peritoneal dialysis (CAPD), which allows continuous dialysis using three to five exchanges of fluid per day via disposable bags.
- Automated peritoneal dialysis (APD), whereby larger volumes of fluid are instilled and drained by the use of a small machine by the bedside, is used when either more intense dialysis is needed or when, for social reasons, the night is the preferred time for treatment.

ABC of Kidney Disease, Second edition.
Edited by David Goldsmith, Satish Jayawardene and Penny Ackland.
© 2013 John Wiley & Sons, Ltd. Published 2013 by John Wiley & Sons, Ltd.

Introduction

Thomas Graham described the founding principles of dialysis over 100 years ago. Even though the first treatments for acute kidney injury (AKI) were performed in the 1920s, chronic dialysis treatment for end stage renal failure (ESRF) did not become a reality until 1960. In the following few years, a series of breakthroughs in both dialysis technology and vascular access enabled chronic renal replacement therapy (RRT) to become established in both the United States and Europe by the mid-1960s. Chronic haemodialysis (HD) became widely available in the United Kingdom in the early 1970s (largely as a home-based therapy), and continuous ambulatory peritoneal dialysis (CAPD) became increasingly popular during the early 1980s. There are now over 2.0 million patients receiving regular dialysis worldwide and around 36,000 in the United Kingdom alone (Box 10.1 and Figure 10.1).

Box 10.1 **Some basic facts about renal replacement therapy in the United Kingdom**

- The most common cause of end-stage renal disease is diabetic nephropathy
- Demand for dialysis will continue to increase over the next 10 years by as much as 150% for HD
- The minimum estimated prevalence of RRT in the United Kingdom at the end of 2003 was 632 patients per million population
- Of new patients, 22% starting RRT are >75 years old and 12% of all prevalent patients are >75 years old
- In 2003, 67.5% of RRT patients received HD and 29.2% PD (3.3% had a transplant)
- The average cost of dialysis is £30 000 per patient per year
- The cost of a kidney transplant is £20 000 per patient per transplant with immunosuppression costs of £6500 per patient per year
- Mortality rate in dialysis patients is about 20% annually
- Commonest cause of death is cardiovascular disease, the risk of which is 30 times higher in dialysis patients than age-matched controls

---

Indications for starting renal replacement therapy

There is relatively little difference in opinion about intractable hyperkalaemia, acidosis, uraemic symptoms (nausea, pruritus,

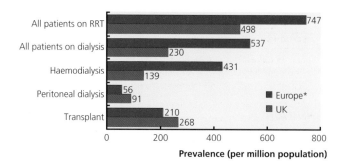

*Germany, Spain, Italy, France and Holland as an average

Figure 10.1 Patient numbers and modalities of treatment in end stage renal failure.

malaise) and therapy-resistant fluid overload being firm indications to commence dialysis. There is, however, wider variation in clinical practice as to when to start a relatively asymptomatic patient. A cut-off based on measured or calculated GFR may be applied. In general, this would be set in the CKD stage 5 range (estimated GFR ~10–15 mL/min). The advantages of such a 'well start' are multiple, and allow for maintenance of health prior to the development of significant abnormalities in either overall function or body composition. Furthermore, it allows dialysis provision to be built up slowly to compensate for further reduction of residual renal function (RRF). There is, however, still no robust (randomized controlled) evidence-base for such an approach. It is important to note that there is considerable variation in the level of GFR individuals may tolerate before becoming markedly uraemic. This may necessitate even earlier starts. The potential price for later initiation is that sudden decompensation may occur, requiring emergency treatment and a 'crash-landing' onto dialysis. This confers a reduction in patient survival that persists for at least the first three years of subsequent therapy.

The general indications for starting dialysis are summarized in Table 10.1.

Table 10.1 Indications for renal replacement therapy.

Acute kidney injury (see Chapter 2)		CKD*	
Hyperkalaemia	K persistently > 6.5. ECG changes	CKD stage 5	eGFR < 15 mL/min
Acidosis	pH < 7.1 resistant to medical therapy	Hyperkalaemia	
Fluid overload	Particularly if compromising lung function	Fluid overload	
Symptomatic uraemia	Pericarditis Neuropathy Encephalopathy	Symptomatic uraemia	
Sepsis and multi-organ failure	Prompt intervention with RRT to prevent uraemic effects on myocardium, clotting and wound healing	Malnutrition	
Poisoning	e.g. lithium, methanol		

*Initiation of RRT in chronic kidney disease varies from unit to unit. Listed are some contributing factors.
CKD, chronic kidney disease; eGFR, estimated glomerular filtration rate; RRT, renal replacement therapy.

Preparation for renal replacement therapy

Timely and effective preparation for RRT, as well as assiduous management of the complications of CKD, is crucial. Optimal therapy while on dialysis will only partially compensate for previous deficiencies in care, with hypertension, functional/structural cardiovascular disease, malnutrition, parathyroid hyperplasia and renal bone disease already being well established in the predialysis phase. There are a number of key issues, covered below, that require a properly configured multidisciplinary team. They need to be delivered in the most effective and appropriate way regarding an individual's social and ethnic sensibilities.

Choice of dialysis modality (see Chapter 4)

Although there may be certain overriding medical or social imperatives, the choice between peritoneal dialysis (PD) and HD (either unit- or home-based) should be free, and not constrained by either clinician's prejudice or resource issues. Sufficient time and information must be provided to allow patients and families to make this choice. Poor or compelled choice will result in a higher chance of treatment failure, and poorer long-term outcomes (therapies are summarized in Table 10.2).

Dialysis access

The vascular access of choice for HD remains the arteriovenous fistula (AVF). This requires the anastomosis of an artery to a suitable segment of vein (usually either at the wrist or in the antecubital fossa). This section of vein receives arterial pressure blood and becomes 'arterialized'. This results in a structure with a thick wall, readily accessible, and with adequate flow within it to sustain an extracorporeal circuit. If there are no suitable peripheral veins, a piece of synthetic material can be inserted (usually a polytetrafluoroethylene, or PTFE, graft) and this is subsequently needled for access. For the reasons of the time taken for the AVF to mature (4–8 weeks), and an initial failure rate, which may be as high as 30% (especially in older, arteriopathic or diabetic patients), this procedure must be performed in good time (Renal NSF recommends six months in advance of likely need). A Tenckhoff catheter for PD, to allow fluid to be instilled into the peritoneal cavity, can be inserted either at laparotomy, laparoscopically or percutaneously, but usually once the decision to start dialysis has been made (Figure 10.2).

Dietary restriction

Specialist dietetic interaction is needed to establish the degree of restriction required in potassium, phosphate, sodium and water intake. The final diet, though, must maintain a reasonable level of protein intake (1 g/kg/day) and avoid malnutrition.

Treatment of anaemia

This may require correction of absolute and/or functional iron deficiency or other haematinics and starting erythropoietin therapy (see Chapter 5).

Table 10.2 Relative advantages and disadvantages of haemo- and peritoneal dialysis.

	Haemodialysis	Peritoneal dialysis
Methods and procedures	Three 4-hour sessions a week, usually in hospital Some flexibility with days and sessions Not reliant on patient's ability to learn or carry out procedures	Continuous dialysis using up to four exchanges/day or cycling at night Procedure done at home and can fit more easily into lifestyle and work Reliant upon patient or other person to perform the procedure safely
Dialysis access	Acute access with venous catheters has high complication rate (infection, stenosis, thrombosis) Fistulae need 2–3 months to mature before use AV fistulae can be difficult to form in patients with vascular disease	Access relatively easy to establish Can be used immediately Comparatively more contraindications (stoma, bowel adhesions, inoperable hernias, obesity)
Fluid balance/ ultrafiltration	Set at the beginning of dialysis and is predictable Amount of fluid to be removed is limited by cardiac function (increased risk of intradialytic hypotension)	Less predictable Controlled by concentration of dextrose (or glucose polymer) in dialysate Integrity of the peritoneum as membrane declines with time, esp. with frequent use of higher dextrose concentrations
Complications	Catheter infections and associated complications (septicaemia, SBE etc.) can be life-threatening Cardiovascular death from arrhythmias, myocardial infarction and stroke are increased IDH predisposes)	Exit site infections are rarely serious and peritonitis, if persistent, usually resolves after removal of catheter Recurrent infections and membrane failure lead to high dropout rate Hernias and leaks from increased peritoneal pressure
Psychosocial considerations	Transport to and from the unit three times a week can disrupt patient and family schedules and prolong dialysis sessions Holidays are hard to plan as patient must rely on local dialysis facilities Body image problems associated with access/fistulae Erectile dysfunction and poor libido	Care of a family member at home can be easier Transport to hospital only needed for clinics or emergencies PD fluids can be delivered worldwide with prior notice Body image problems associated with PD catheter Erectile dysfunction and poor libido

AV, arteriovenous; PD, peritoneal dialysis; SBE, subacute bacterial endocarditis; IDH, intradialytic hypotension.

Psychosocial issues (see Chapter 4)

Support for both the patient and their family is required for the psychological impact of RRT, and practical guidance from a specialist social worker into the benefits etc. that are available if work becomes problematic. Sexual function is often affected, with problems with both libido and erectile dysfunction (amenable to the conventional range of interventions). Although fertility in women of child-bearing age is impaired, effective contraception is essential due to the immense problems associated with pregnancy while on dialysis. These risks are largely normalized by successful transplantation.

Renal replacement therapy

Haemodialysis

HD involves circulating blood through a disposable dialyser. This contains hollow fibres of a selectively permeable material, giving a large total surface area ($1–2 \, m^2$). Dialysate is produced by the continuous combination of concentrate with highly treated tap water (microbiologically pure, low endotoxin concentration and depleted in minerals). This flows around the hollow fibres in the opposite direction to blood. It contains a low concentration of factors to be removed and a higher concentration of bicarbonate, allowing diffusion into the blood and correction of acidosis. Removal of accumulated fluid is achieved by applying a pressure gradient across the dialysis membrane, resulting in controlled ultrafiltration (Figure 10.3).

Conventionally, heparin is used to prevent clotting and the treatment is performed three times a week, for 3–5 h per session. This results in adequate control of biochemistry (though not normalized), fluid overload, acidosis and uraemic symptoms in *most* patients.

Peritoneal dialysis

This technique involves using the peritoneum as the dialysis membrane. Pre-packaged fluid is instilled into the peritoneal space. It is allowed to dwell for a period of time. Waste products to be removed diffuse from the blood into the fluid. Again, the dialysate contains factors that do not need to be removed at similar concentrations to normal plasma (calcium, magnesium, sodium etc.). Acidosis is corrected by the diffusion of buffer from the fluid into the blood, and ultrafiltration occurs down an oncotic gradient. This is produced by the fluid having a higher osmolality than plasma (due to a high concentration of glucose or glucose polymer within the instilled fluid).

Ready drainage relies on good tube placement and function. The most common cause of failure is constipation with tube displacement, or inspissation of omental fat into the catheter's multiple distal perforations. PD patients characteristically are prescribed aperients to ideally promote two soft bowel motions per day. The main limitations of the technique relate to the development of peritonitis, resulting from either an infected exit site, poor adherence to the technical challenges associated with PD bag changes or bacterial translocation across the bowel wall.

There are a number of refinements of the PD method. CAPD involves 3–5 exchanges of fluid per day, every day (due to the intrinsically lower solute removal efficiency compared with HD). The patient performs these manually, with the bag being disconnected between each exchange.

In some patients, either more intensive dialysis is needed or, for social reasons, the night is the preferred time for the treatment to take place. In this setting, automated peritoneal dialysis (APD) can be used. This allows larger volumes to be instilled and drained by

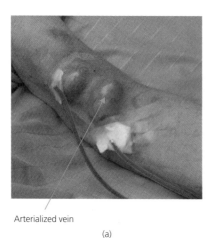

Arterialized vein

(a)

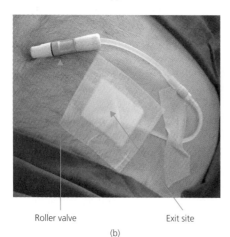

Roller valve   Exit site

(b)

Figure 10.2 (a) Arteriovenous fistula. (b) Tenckhoff (peritoneal dialysis) catheter.

the use of a small machine by the bedside (Figure 10.4). Assisted APD is a method by which patients can undergo APD at home either while they are waiting to be trained or if they are unable to do the dialysis themselves. It does have cost implications but offers great benefits to patients. A paid carer visits once a day to strip and prepare the APD machine for the next dialysis. The patient or a family member will perform the connection at night and disconnection the next morning. The carer may also perform blood pressure (BP) monitoring and/or exit site dressing.

Up until recently, the composition of all PD fluids was very similar. Glucose was used to produce the oncotic gradient and lactate was used as buffer (absorbed and converted to bicarbonate by the liver). Due to the limitations of using these compounds, and an increasing appreciation of the biological toxicities of glucose degradation products, a number of other fluids have subsequently been developed with a greater degree of biocompatibility (summarized in Table 10.3).

Monitoring adequacy of renal replacement therapy

The aim of chronic dialysis therapy is to replicate as far as possible the normal functions of the failed kidney(s). Patients are monitored, usually monthly, for a wide range of indices relating to solute clearance, mineral metabolism, volume status, nutrition and anaemia (summarized in Table 10.4).

Solute clearance

This is usually measured as small solute clearance, and the conventional marker is urea. Clearance is measured by blood sampling before and after HD, or with a combination of blood samples and samples of waste fluid in PD. A variety of mathematical treatments

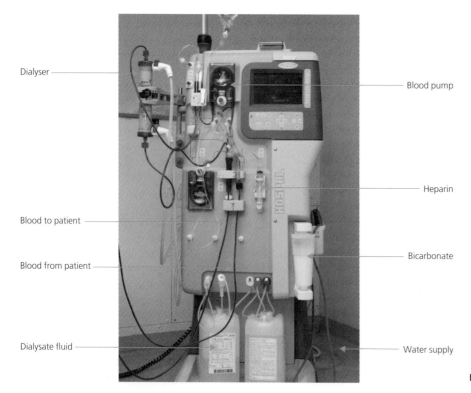

Dialyser

Blood to patient

Blood from patient

Dialysate fluid

Blood pump

Heparin

Bicarbonate

Water supply

Figure 10.3 Haemodialysis machine.

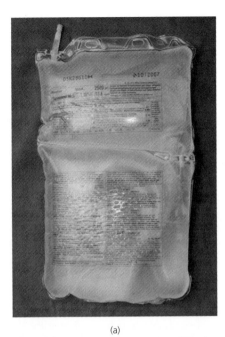

(a)

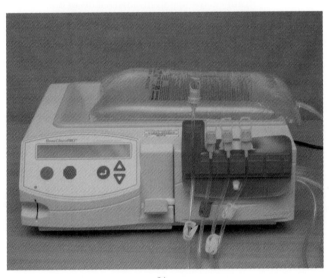

(b)

Figure 10.4 (a) Peritoneal dialysate fluid. (b) Automated peritoneal dialysis machine.

Table 10.3 Types of peritoneal dialysate fluids.

Fluid type	Comments
Conventional lactate buffered glucose-based solutions	Fluid removal is dependent on glucose concentration. Low biocompatibility and high glucose degradation products.
Bicarbonate-based buffered solutions	Uses bicarbonate alone or in combination with lactate. This has been shown to reduce pain during infusion and may improve long-term preservation of the peritoneal membrane.
Glucose polymer solutions (icodextrin)	Contains a glucose polymer less likely to be absorbed into the body. Also benefits long-term PD patients with poor ultrafiltration. It is used once each day for the long dwell. Use reduces systemic glucose exposure.
Amino-acid-containing solutions	Contains amino acids instead of glucose. Possibly useful for patients with malnutrition and hypoalbuminaemia. More than once daily use may result in acidosis.

Table 10.4 Treatment aims for dialysis patients.

Factor	Aims
Haemoglobin	10.5–12.5 g/dL
Potassium	HD: 3.5–6.5 mmol/L
	PD: 3.3–5.5 mmol/L
Calcium	Normal range
Parathyroid hormone	2–4 × normal range
Phosphate	1.2–1.7 mmol/L
Albumin	Normal range
Systolic BP	$\leq$140 mmHg predialysis
Diastolic BP	$\leq$90 mmHg predialysis
Adequacy	HD: Kt/V $\geq$ 1.2
	PD: Kt/V $\geq$ 1.7 ($\geq$2.0 for APD)

APD, automated peritoneal dialysis; PD, peritoneal dialysis; HD, haemodialysis; BP, blood pressure.

Table 10.5 Monitoring fluid balance.

Situation	Effects
Dehydrated	Weight loss, dizziness, nausea, constipation, hypotension, cramps
Ideal weight	Nil
Fluid overloaded	Weight increases, feet/ankles swell, breathlessness, hypertension

are applied to these measurements and the adequacy of clearance calculated. Failure to reach certain thresholds is associated with increasing symptoms, failure to thrive and increased mortality. In HD, dialyser size, blood flow through the dialyser, access quality and treatment time can all be modulated to enhance clearance. In PD the dialysate volumes, number of exchanges, dwell time and use of APD are the main factors that can be altered to vary the efficiency of dialysis. The clearance of other factors can be measured (middle molecules) and these may influence the development of some long-term complications.

Maintenance of dry/desired weight

This refers to the patient's weight best replicating the normal level of hydration (Table 10.5) and is important in managing hypertension

and preventing the development of left ventricular hypertrophy and cardiac failure.

Residual renal function

Maintenance of RRF reduces mortality and facilitates volume management, while avoiding the draconian fluid restriction required in anephric patients (500–750 mL/day). Nonsteroidal anti-inflammatory drug (NSAID) usage may reduce RRF, and therefore continued caution is required even in patients established on RRT.

Mineral metabolism and renal bone disease

This requires careful modulation of phosphate binders (type and dose), vitamin D and calcimimetics/parathyroidectomy.

Table 10.6 Complications of dialysis.

Haemodialysis	Peritoneal dialysis
Hypertension	
Increased cardiovascular risk	
Malnutrition	
Renal bone disease	
Anaemia	
Psychosocial/sexual factors	
Intradialytic hypotension	Hernias
Adverse dialysis-related symptoms (cramps, headache etc.)	Fluid leaks
Access issues (infection, aneurysm, thrombosis and rupture)	Peritonitis (+subsequent membrane/ultrafiltration failure)
Amyloid	

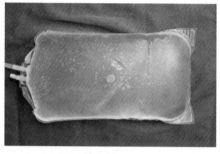

(a)

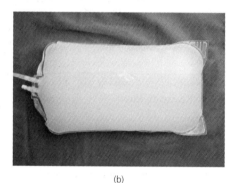

(b)

Figure 10.5 Drained fluid in peritoneal dialysis peritonitis. (a) Normal peritoneal dialysate drainage. (b) Cloudy dialysate drainage in peritonitis.

Other factors

These include assessment of suitability for transplantation and monitoring of complications (Table 10.6 and Figure 10.5).

Developments in delivery of renal replacement therapy

PD continues to be an important treatment modality, both in the United Kingdom and Holland – two European countries with socialized healthcare systems and chronic underfunding of HD

facilities – and in particular across the developing world. In the United Kingdom, the National Institute for Health and Clinical Excellence (NICE) published clinical guidelines in 2011 on PD particularly recommending it for patients who have RRF, all children under two years of age and adults without significant associated comorbidities. Wholesale adoption of the newer and more expensive PD solutions is currently being handicapped by the lack of appropriate outcome studies, although they do seem to have a wide range of benefits in terms of peritoneal function, systemic biocompatibility and cardiovascular response.

HD technology is also becoming more complex, with the use of biosensors to detect the physiological response to treatment and run biofeedback systems to improve treatment tolerability. Perturbations of dialysate temperature and sodium concentration, as well as adding a degree of convective clearance to dialysis, can ameliorate the common problem of intradialytic hypotension (IDH). These technologies, however, are largely adaptive to compensate for the high ultrafiltration rates and short treatment times driven by current pressures on dialysis resources. Increasing interest is occurring in daily dialysis (short hours during the day, or long, low-efficiency treatment overnight) in either a unit- or home-based environment.

There is a resurgence of interest in home-based HD, with improvements in water preparation and machine portability, and the increasing realization that with long overnight (quotidian) dialysis, or daily short-session dialysis, there can be very significant improvements in anaemia, calcium–phosphate balance, acidosis, nutrition, BP, lipid profiles and left ventricular hypertrophy compared to 'standard' thrice-weekly, four-hour sessions.

It is certain that the escalating numbers of patients on treatment and increasing comorbidity load will require continued refinement of RRT, while not replacing the need for early identification and assiduous preparation mentally and physically in the predialysis phase.

Further reading

Bender FH, Bernardini J, Piraino B (2006) Prevention of infectious complications in peritoneal dialysis: Best demonstrated practices. *Kidney Int Suppl* **70**(103): S44–54.

Greneche S, D'Andon A, Jacquelinet C *et al.* (2005) Choosing between peritoneal dialysis and haemodialysis: A critical appraisal of the literature. *Nephrol Ther* **1**(4): 213–220.

Hayashi R, Huang E, Nissenson AR (2006) Vascular access for hemodialysis. *Nat Clin Pract Nephrol* **2**(9): 504–13.

Light P (2006) Current understanding of optimal blood pressure goals in dialysis patients. *Curr Hypertens Rep* **8**(5):413–419.

NHS Information National Library for Kidney Disease, www.library.nhs.uk/kidney.

Rabindranath KS, Strippoli GF, Daly C *et al.* (2006) Haemodiafiltration, haemofiltration and haemodialysis for end-stage kidney disease. *Cochrane Database Syst Rev* **18**(4): CD006258.

CHAPTER 11

Renal Transplantation

Ming He and John Taylor

Guy's and St Thomas' NHS Foundation Trust, London, UK

OVERVIEW

- Kidney transplantation is generally the optimal form of renal replacement therapy (RRT) in terms of patient survival, quality of life and cost-effectiveness.

- Immunosuppressive treatment is necessary for the life of the kidney transplant – hence compliance is a major issue in the graft survival.

- (Blood group) ABO compatibility is desirable between the donor and recipient. The risk of transplant rejection is less where there is good human leukocyte antigen (HLA) antigen 'match'. Blood transfusions can sensitize the recipient to potential donor HLA antigens, and so should be avoided if possible when there is a likelihood of transplantation.

- A live, unrelated transplant with complete HLA mismatching has a better long-term outcome than a cadaveric organ with no mismatch at all.

- Living donors now account for > 25% of all kidneys transplanted in the United Kingdom, and this is increasing.

- Post-operatively, most kidneys function immediately. Acute tubular necrosis (ATN) is the single most likely cause of delayed graft function, and is usually reversible.

- The main complications of kidney transplantation are:
  - Rejection: 10–30% of transplanted kidneys are acutely rejected; this presents as a decline in renal function usually within the first three months. Hyperacute rejection, which occurs within hours, is very rare.
  - Tubulo-interstital fibrosis, scarring, sclerosis and vasculopathy: this is the main cause of graft failure; progressive and irreversible increases in creatinine, associated with proteinuria, usually occur over years.
  - Infection: the main concern is susceptibility to opportunistic infections, notably *Cytomegalovirus* and *Pneumocystis carinii*.
  - Malignancy: increased risk of post-transplantation lymphoproliferative disorders associated with Epstein–Barr virus infection.
  - Recurrence: all forms of glomerulonephritis can recur and affect the transplanted kidney.

- Graft survival at one year is now approximately 90–95% for cadaveric kidneys and more than 95% for kidneys from living donors. Overall, graft survival is about 50% at 10 years; the main causes of graft attrition are either tubulo-interstital fibrosis, scarring, sclerosis and vasculopathy or death of the patient.

Introduction

Kidney transplantation is the optimal form of renal replacement therapy (RRT), whether in terms of patient survival, quality of life or cost-effectiveness. However, this option is available to only about 30% of RRT patients. The number of patients on the waiting list is increasing as transplantation is now a well-established procedure (Figure 11.1), immunosuppression regimes are continually refined and previously contraindicated recipients are now included (e.g. HIV-positive patients). Equally, tissue-typing and blood group incompatibilities are now more easily circumvented, and there has been a significant change in the type of kidney donations now accepted, for example altruistic.

As well as kidney transplantation alone, kidneys can be transplanted at the same time as a liver (e.g. cirrhosis with kidney failure, or primary hyperoxaluria) or a heart. Simultaneous kidney–pancreas transplantation is less common, but a significant treatment option for type 1 diabetic patients with end stage renal failure (ESRF) (Figure 11.2). Space considerations preclude more detailed descriptions.

Immunological aspects of transplantation

The almost universal need to continue immunosuppressive treatment for the life of the kidney transplant for all donor/recipient combinations means that compliance is a major issue in graft survival.

Acquired immunity consists of the cellular (T-cell mediated) and humoral (B-cell mediated) responses, and both are involved in graft rejection. Essentially, the acquired immune response depends on recognition of graft antigens as being foreign and this stimulates various effector mechanisms against the graft, such as macrophage activation, natural killer cell response, delayed hypersensitivity, cellular cytotoxicity, plus complement fixation.

ABC of Kidney Disease, Second edition.
Edited by David Goldsmith, Satish Jayawardene and Penny Ackland.
© 2013 John Wiley & Sons, Ltd. Published 2013 by John Wiley & Sons, Ltd.

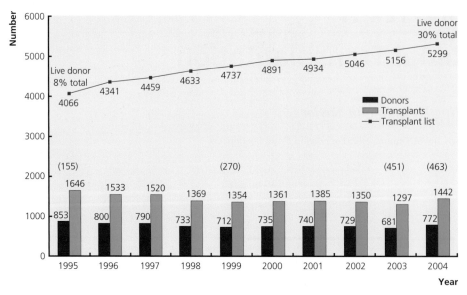

Figure 11.1 Cadaveric kidney programme in the United Kingdom, 1995–2004. Number of donors, transplants and patients on the active transplant list at 31 December each year (live donors indicated in parentheses). (*Source:* Figures from United Kingdom Transplant (UKT).)

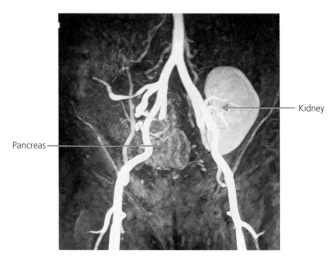

Figure 11.2 Magnetic resonance angiogram showing a kidney transplant on the right and a pancreas transplant on the left of the figure.

Figures 11.3 and 11.4 detail the immunological barriers to transplantation, and 'matching' – the extreme polymorphism of alleles at the human leukocyte antigen (HLA) loci mean that a degree of mismatch is likely between donor and recipient, and this is usually expressed as a mismatch score, i.e. 0–0–0 being a perfect match and 2–2–2 being a complete mismatch.

The kidney donor

There are two broad categories: cadaveric or living. Cadaveric donors are either heart-beating or non-heart-beating donors (NHBDs). Table 11.1 shows contraindications to cadaveric kidney donation. There were over 18.5 million people on the UK Organ Donor Register in January 2012.

Cadaveric

The largest group of transplants comes from brain-stem dead patients with maintained cardiac output, usually in an intensive therapy unit (ITU) setting. Cause of death is usually intracranial haemorrhage or trauma. Kidneys from NHBDs, i.e. post-circulatory arrest, have shown comparable rates of success. However, the drawback to this approach is the warm ischaemic time (the time between cessation of heartbeat with the diagnosis of death and cooling of the organ). Of all potential donors in the ITU setting, consent for donation is not forthcoming from 36% of families.

Once a donor is identified, HLA typing is carried out and the most suitable recipient found through a national matching scheme administered by the NHS Blood and Transplant Authority (see website in Further reading). Clinically, peri-retrieval factors such as haemodynamic instability, ventilation, hypothermia and diabetes insipidus are managed to optimize perfusion.

Living

This now accounts for 25–30% of all kidneys transplanted in the United Kingdom (Figure 11.1), and in some Scandinavian and American centres live transplants are more numerous than deceased donor options. Living donation is on the increase in the United Kingdom – it may become the most practical way to address the donor organ deficit for kidneys at least, especially as live-unrelated donation (e.g. between spouses or altruistic) is yielding excellent outcomes and newer surgical techniques are being employed with the benefits of reduced pain, greater cosmesis and faster postoperative recovery (e.g. laparoscopic nephrectomy). A live-unrelated transplant with complete HLA mismatching still has a better long-term outcome than a cadaveric organ with no mismatch at all (Figure 11.3). Another advantage of living donors is the possibility of considering a 'marginal' recipient who may not be suitable for a cadaveric kidney.

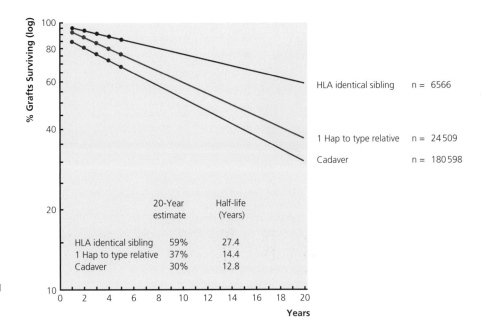

Figure 11.3 Relationship between survival and type of donor (first kidney transplants 1985–2004). (CTS-K-1503-0206).

The process of evaluation of the living donor is outlined fully in the Living Donor Guidelines, as set by the British Transplant Society and UK Renal Association. Patients and potential donors

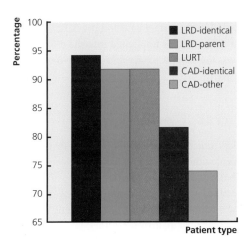

Figure 11.4 Three-year renal graft survival. UCLA data 28 945 patients. The outcome of HLA-identical cadaveric kidneys is inferior to all categories of live donor, including living unrelated transplants. CAD: cadaveric donor; LRD: living-related donor; LURD: living unrelated donor. (*Source:* Terasaki PI *et al.* (1995) High survival rates of kidney transplants from spousal and living unrelated donors. *New Engl J Medi* **333**(6): 333–6.)

Table 11.1 Contraindications to cadaveric donation.

Absolute	Relative
Chronic renal disease	Age < 5 or > 60
Potentially metastasizing malignancy	Mild hypertension
Severe hypertension	Treated infection
Bacterial septicaemia	Nonoliguric acute tubular necrosis
Current intravenous drug user	Positive hepatitis B and C serology
HIV positive	Intestinal perforation with spillage
Warm ischaemia > 45 min	Prolonged cold ischaemia
Irreversible acute kidney injury	High-risk behaviour

are given information leaflets and videos, and donors undergo a full series of screening investigations. Those who go on to donate have a risk of death of 1 in 3000, and there is no excess risk of hypertension or ESRF post-donation. Regardless, monitoring of blood pressure, urinary protein excretion and renal function in the longer term in kidney donors are important. However, the final donation rate may be as low as 20–25% in all those who are assessed as potential live donors. The reasons for this vary from immunological (40%) and medical (20%), to donor withdrawal or uncertainty (up to 40%). All potential living donors (whether related or unrelated) are assessed independently at a local level to determine their suitability for donation under terms set out by the Human Tissue Act 2004. More complex cases can be referred to the Human Tissue Authority. See http://www.uktransplant.org.uk/ukt/how_to_become_a_donor/living_kidney_donation/questions_and_answers.jsp.

Recipient

Kidney transplantation is considered suitable for patients with chronic kidney disease requiring dialysis or predicted to require dialysis within 6 to 12 months. In the United Kingdom, around 25% of such patients are transplanted, the main constraint being donor supply. The main principles to consider during recipient selection are:

- the benefits in terms of quality and duration of life should outweigh the risks to the patient in terms of the procedure and subsequent immunosuppression, especially in patients with other comorbidities or older patients;
- with cadaveric organs, justifying the use of a limited resource and allocation should be in terms of maximum benefit to society (patients not likely to survive five years or less should not receive a cadaveric donor kidney);
- in living donors, the risk to the donor should be justified by the predicted benefit of a successful transplant.

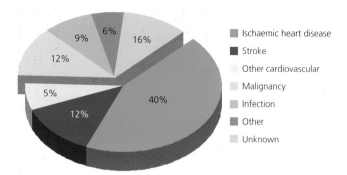

Figure 11.5 Cardiovascular disease is the major cause of death with a functioning graft in renal transplant recipients. First grafts 1984–1996 92 deaths in 1260 patients. (*Source:* Kavanagh D *et al.* (1999) Electrocardiogram and outcome following renal transplantation. *Nephron* **81**(1): 109–10.)

Apart from these general issues and those pertaining to the undertaking of major surgical intervention in the context of renal disease, various specific clinical factors must be considered.

Infection

Active infections should be eradicated where possible (e.g. tuberculosis); patients with chronic hepatitis B or C can prove challenging, as post-transplantation exacerbation of virally driven liver pathology is well recognized. Patients with recurrent urinary tract infection are considered for native nephrectomy. Those at risk of post-transplant tuberculosis (TB) should have TB prophylaxis post-operatively.

Malignancy

Patients with current malignancy are not considered for transplantation, but treated patients may be transplanted after a recurrence-free period, depending on type of malignancy.

Cardiovascular disease

As this is the most common cause of death (and hence graft loss) post-transplant (Figure 11.5), any history or evidence of disease is thoroughly investigated and treated as appropriate. In addition, certain groups of asymptomatic patients, such as those aged over 50 years, smokers and all diabetics, should undergo cardiovascular screening (e.g. stress echocardiography, nuclear scintigraphy, coronary angiography, iliac arterial imaging).

Bladder function

Urological problems (e.g. outflow obstruction) should be investigated before transplantation.

Surgical aspects

Donor/retrieval

Cadaveric kidneys usually come from multi-organ retrievals and are shipped on ice. The timing of the recipient transplant is set to minimize the cold ischaemic time. The shorter this is, the more likely the immediate function of the kidney, which has a positive effect on graft outcome.

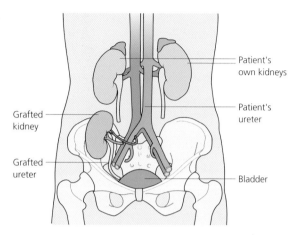

Figure 11.6 Grafted kidney placed heterotopically in the iliac fossa.

Living donors can be operated on electively, for instance timed to 'pre-empt' the need for dialysis.

Recipient

The graft is usually placed heterotopically in the iliac fossa (Figure 11.6), which is extraperitoneal in adults but is placed intraperitoneally in a child weighing less than 20 kg. The iliac vessels are used in the former case and the aorta/inferior vena cava in the latter. The ureter is implanted into the dome of the bladder. In the pelvis, the kidney is safe and there are no restrictions on recipient activity.

Post-operative management

Most kidneys function immediately – certainly those from living donors almost without fail. Immediate post-operative concerns are with fluid balance and risk of bleeding.

Deterioration in kidney function may be reversible (hypovolaemia, acute tubular necrosis (ATN), ureteric obstruction, drug toxicity especially calcineurin inhibitors, acute rejection) or irreversible (hyperacute rejection, vascular thrombosis). Ultrasound with Doppler assessment of blood flow and percutaneous biopsy should help identify these causes (Figure 11.7).

ATN is the single most likely cause of delayed graft function and tends to occur in cadaveric kidneys, especially those from older donors and kidneys with a prolonged cold ischaemic time or from NHBDs. Dialysis is required until the ATN resolves.

Immunosuppression

Immunosuppression is initiated at the time of transplant. There are various classes of immunosuppressive agents (Table 11.2), used in combination to prevent rejection and minimize dose-related side-effects (Table 11.3 and Figure 11.8). Different agents may also be used during different phases of immunosuppressive therapy, namely induction, maintenance and treatment of rejection episodes.

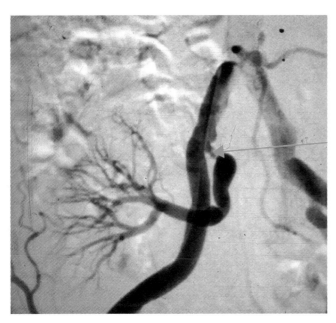

Figure 11.7 Renal transplant angiogram showing a 95% stenosis in the transplant artery (see arrow).

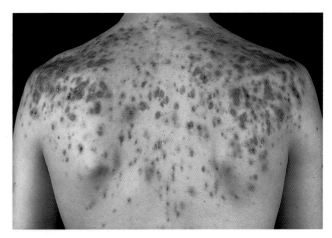

Figure 11.8 Severe acne due to steroids.

Complications

There may be complications related to surgery (as discussed briefly above) or longer-term problems related to rejection, infection, malignancy and recurrence of the original disease – all of which have an impact on the overall outcome or success of the procedure. There is also a risk of mortality, especially during the first 100 post-operative days (Figure 11.9).

Rejection

Hyperacute rejection occurs within hours and is extremely rare. It results from the presence of pre-existing antibodies in the recipient to donor antigens. There is no effective treatment and the graft must be removed. Prevention depends on ABO matching and pre-transplant lymphocyte cross-matching.

Acute rejection occurs in 10–30% of recipients with current immunosuppressive protocols, and presents as an early decline in renal function, i.e. within the first three months. It is confirmed by percutaneous needle renal biopsy and treated with high-dose steroids and some modification of the maintenance immunosuppressive regimen. Due to the need for significant and sustained surveillance of renal transplant patients (regular renal function testing), we generally recommend waiting for 12 months

Table 11.2 Classes of immunosuppressive drugs.

Corticosteroids	Broad anti-inflammatory and immunosuppressive effects; inhibit activation of T-cells. Started at transplantation with weaning off after a few months as there are numerous long-term side-effects.
Antiproliferative agents (e.g. azathioprine, MMF)	Inhibits purine metabolism and DNA synthesis. Used in suppressing rejection, MMF more potent.
Calcineurin inhibitors (e.g. ciclosporin, tacrolimus)	Block the intracellular signalling pathway leading to IL-2 release and amplification of immune response. Narrow therapeutic index, requires regular blood level monitoring. Tacrolimus is more potent.
Cell cycle inhibitors (e.g. sirolimus)	Prevents proliferation of T-cells, more potent than ciclosporin but not nephrotoxic. Reduces the incidence of acute rejection.
Biological agents (e.g. OKT3, basiliximab, daclizimab, ALG, ATG)	Monoclonal antibodies targeting CD3 or the IL-2 receptor have a role in the treatment of acute rejection. They are associated with cytokine release syndrome. IL-2 receptor antagonist given at induction reduces acute rejection.

MMF, mycophenolate mofetil.

Table 11.3 Principal side-effects of immunosuppressive therapy.

Corticosteroids	Ciclosporin	Tacrolimus	Azathioprine	Mycophenolate mofetil	Sirolimus
Hypertension	Nephrotoxic effects	Nephrotoxic effects	Marrow suppression	Diarrhoea/gastrointestinal upset	Dyslipidaemia
Glucose intolerance	Hypertension	Hypertension		Marrow suppression	Marrow suppression
Dyslipidaemia	Glucose intolerance	Glucose intolerance			Acne
Osteoporosis	Dyslipidaemia	Dyslipidaemia			Poor wound healing
	Gum hyperplasia	Alopecia			
	Hirsutism				

Source: Modified from Denton MD *et al.* (1999) Immunosuppressive strategies in transplantation. *Lancet* **353**: 1083–91.

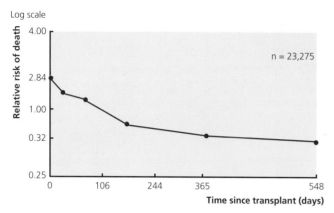

Log scale

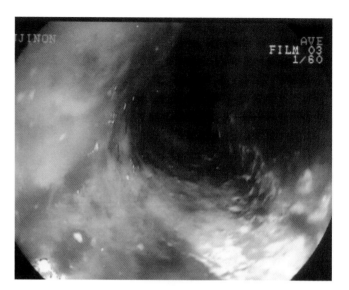

Figure 11.9 Survival benefit of renal transplantation. (*Source:* Adapted from Wolfe RA *et al.* (1999) Comparison of mortality in all patients on dialysis, patients on dialysis awaiting transplantation, and recipients of a first cadaveric transplant. *New Engl J Medi* **341**(23): 1725–30.)

Figure 11.11 Oesophageal ulcer and slough due to candida.

post-transplantation before sanctioning pregnancy or extended foreign travel.

Late acute rejection is one feature of poor concordance with therapy.

Chronic allograft nephropathy

This is the main cause of graft failure. Both immunological (incidence of acute rejection, degree of HLA mismatch) and non-immunological factors (hypertension, diabetes mellitus, hyperlipidaemia and chronic exposure to calcineurin inhibitors) are involved. A progressive, irreversible loss of renal function is seen, particularly when associated with proteinuria. Figure 11.10 shows histopathological changes associated with tubulo-interstital fibrosis, scarring, sclerosis and vasculopathy (formerly known as chronic allograft nephropathy (CAN)). This can be driven by chronic antibody-mediated rejection (i.e. immunological reasons) or by other factors, including calcineurin inhibitor use.

Infection

In the immediate post-operative period, bacterial infections can complicate recovery as in any surgical procedure (e.g. wound, chest, urinary tract). However, the main concern with transplant recipients is the susceptibility to opportunistic infections due to immunosuppressive therapy (Figures 11.11 and 11.12).

Cytomegalovirus is a particular concern in a seropositive to -negative transplant (Figure 11.13), and these recipients should have routine oral prophylaxis with valganciclovir for 90 days. An

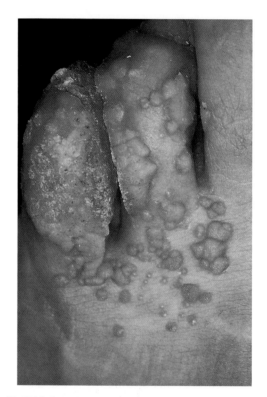

Figure 11.12 Viral warts.

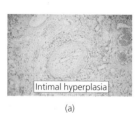
(a)

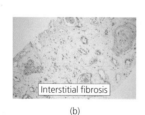
(b)

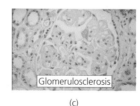
(c)

Figure 11.10 Histology of chronic allograft nephropath: extracellular matrix deposition. (a) Intimal hyperplasia. (b) Interstitial fibrosis. (c) Glomerulosclerosis.

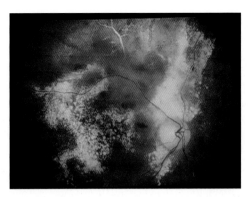

Figure 11.13 Retinal cytomegalovirus infection.

alternative may be regular screening of blood for CMV DNA by polymerase chain reaction techniques. Viral infections may also be involved in malignancies.

Post engraftment, prophylaxis with co-trimoxazole for *Pneumocystis carinii* is given for three months. High-risk patients can receive isoniazid and pyroxidine for TB prophylaxis for six months.

Malignancy

There is a significantly increased risk for lymphoproliferative disorders post-transplantation (PTLD), which is associated with Epstein–Barr virus infection. Treatment of PTLD involves careful reduction or withdrawal of immunosuppression and starting chemotherapy regimens as appropriate.

Skin malignancies, such as squamous cell carcinoma, Kaposi's sarcoma and others with a viral aetiology (e.g. human papilloma virus-related) are also much increased (Figure 11.14).

Recurrence

All forms of glomerulonephritis (IgA nephropathy, familial haemolytic-uraemic syndrome) and some metabolic or systemic diseases (e.g. diabetes, amyloidosis) can recur after transplantation; despite this, the contribution of this cause of total loss of allograft function is small. In some unlucky individuals, disease recurrence

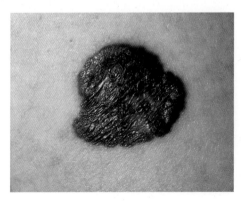

Figure 11.14 Malignant melanoma.

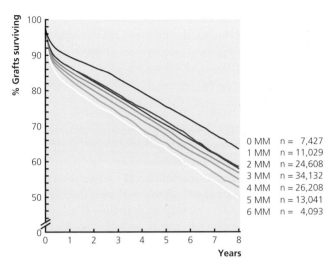

Figure 11.15 HLA-A+B+DR Mismatches (first cadaver kidney transplants 1985–2004). (CTS-K-21101-0206).

is a feature of successive transplants. It is rarely possible to effectively treat post-transplantation disease recurrence.

Outcome

Graft survival at one year is approximately 85–90% for cadaveric kidneys and more than 95% for living donors. The attrition rate continues at a steady 3–5% per year (Figure 11.15), so graft survival is about 50% at 10 years overall – hence many patients return to dialysis after 10 years or have a repeat transplant. The main causes of graft attrition are chronic allograft fibrosis and death (usually from cardiac problems). Improvements in graft survival will probably depend on an improved understanding of progressive fibrosis and directed therapies to prevent it, and accurate identification and treatment of those patients with significant cardiac comorbidity.

Living donation is associated with better graft and patient outcomes in general. It also makes pre-emptive renal transplantation more feasible, which is associated with better outcomes.

Compliance/concordance

Graft survival inevitably depends on compliance with immunosuppressive regimens, and non-concordance is a major risk factor in both acute rejection and tubulo-interstital fibrosis, scarring, sclerosis and vasculopathy. Patients with a history of psychosocial problems, such as drug addiction, should be fully assessed and rehabilitated before being entered onto the transplant waiting list.

The future

There are a number of strategies to increase the quantity of organs available for donation in the near future; one of the most feasible is to increase living donation. Widening patient and public awareness from the level of the clinician to national educational campaigns could help with this. More specifically, new legislation (Human

Tissue Act 2004) that came onto the statute book in September 2006 now permits altruistic donation, and 'organ-swapping' within two or more donor–patient pairs who had greater reciprocal HLA matching, i.e. paired or pooled donation.

Major advances using anti-CD 20 antibody plasmapheresis or immunoabsorption now permit successful kidney transplantation even across some ABO blood group compatibilities and in the presence of anti-HLA antibodies (i.e. sensitized patients). Results are not yet as good as seen in less challenging situations, but this for many is still a better option than remaining on dialysis.

Many of the current immunologically active pharmaceutical agents are imprecise and difficult to use. There is much excitement about, and anticipation of, the new generation of more precisely targeted immunological tolerance-permitting drugs, which may be permissive of long-term accommodation, reducing the need for long-term use of potentially nephro- and cardiotoxic medications such as steroids or calcineurin inhibitors.

Xenotransplantation has been considered since the last decade but is not a practicable option at present – not least due to immune incompatibility. This will remain, just as is the case for transplantation immunological tolerance, the future for organ transplantation.

Further reading

British Transplantation Society/The Renal Association. *United Kingdom Guidelines for Living Donor Kidney Transplantation.* Available at http://www.bts.org.uk.

EBPG Expert Group on Renal Transplantation (2002) European best practice guidelines for renal transplantation: Section IV: Long-term management of the transplant recipient. IV.5.1. Cardiovascular risks. Cardiovascular disease after renal transplantation. *Nephrol Dial and Transplant* 17(Suppl 4): 24–5.

Human Tissue Authority website. Available at http://www.hta.gov.uk.

Karlberg I, Nyberg G (1995) Cost-effectiveness studies of renal transplantation. *Int J Tech Assess Health Care* 11: 611–22.

Laupacis A, Keown P, Pus N *et al.* (1996) A study of the quality of life and cost utility of renal transplantation. *Kid Int* 50: 235–42.

Murray JE, Merrill JP, Harrison JH (1955) Renal homotransplantation in identical twins. *Surgical Forum* VI: 432–6.

Wolfe RA, Ashby, VB, Milford EL *et al.* (1999) Comparison of mortality in all patients on dialysis awaiting transplantation, and recipients of a first cadaveric transplant. *New Engl J Medi* 341: 1725–30.

United Kingdom Blood and Transplant, http://www.uktransplant.org.uk/ukt/.

http://www.uktransplant.org.uk/ukt/how_to_become_a_donor/living_kidney_donation/questions_and_answers.jsp.

http://www.kidney.org.uk/Medical-Info/transplant.html.

http://www.dh.gov.uk/assetRoot/04/10/36/86/04103686.pdf.

http://www.uktransplant.org.uk/ukt/about_transplants/legislation/legislation.jsp.

CHAPTER 12

Chronic Kidney Disease, Dialysis and Transplantation in Children

Judy Taylor and Christopher Reid

Guy's and St Thomas' NHS Foundation Trust, London, UK

OVERVIEW

Congenital and structural renal disease

- Antenatal ultrasound scanning during pregnancy detects a range of structural renal abnormalities which require assessment and follow-up during infancy.
- Urinary tract infection (UTI) is commoner in infants and children with certain structural abnormalities of the urinary tract.
- Congenital renal dysplasia is the commonest cause of renal failure in childhood.
- Genetically inherited renal diseases are most likely to present in childhood. These include autosomal recessive polycystic kidney disease, Alport's syndrome and several rare tubular and metabolic disorders.

Childhood nephrotic syndrome

- In nephrotic syndrome, the glomeruli allow small proteins such as albumin to leak out into the urine.
- Childhood nephrotic syndrome commonly occurs between the ages of 1 and 5 years, in boys more often than in girls.
- The majority of children (80–85%) are responsive to steroid treatment, though many of these will have a relapsing course. Other immunosuppressive therapy may be indicated in children who relapse frequently, to minimize the side-effects of steroids.
- Most children 'outgrow' nephrotic syndrome by their late teens without permanent damage to their kidneys, and have an excellent long-term prognosis.
- Renal biopsy is normally reserved for those who do not respond to steroid treatment. In these children, focal segmental glomerulosclerosis is the commonest histological diagnosis with a much poorer prognosis.

Glomerulonephritis

- Glomerulonephritis (GN) is an inflammation of the glomeruli and may be temporary and reversible, or it may progress of chronic kidney disease (CKD). It is usually manifest by raised blood pressure, non-visible haematuria, proteinuria and renal impairment.
- Acute post-streptococcal GN is the commonest cause, with an excellent prognosis for recovery.
- Henoch–Schönlein purpura (HSP) is frequently associated with renal involvement, though this is usually clinically mild and self-limiting. A minority may develop severe GN.
- Haemolytic uraemic syndrome (HUS) is the commonest cause of acute kidney injury (AKI) in childhood. Full recovery is usual when associated with *E. coli* 0157:H7 enterocolitis and diarrhoea.

Renal replacement therapy

- In infants with renal failure, difficult vascular access and inherent cardiovascular instability mean that peritoneal dialysis, as opposed to haemodialysis (HD), is usually the modality of choice.
- Transplantation (usually possible from around 2 years of age) offers the best quality of life even though regrafting is probably inevitable at some stage.
- Living related donor transplantation is increasingly undertaken in most paediatric centres, and this facilitates pre-emptive transplantation whereby dialysis is avoided.

Introduction

Although many of the principles governing kidney disease management are common to adults and children, the underlying disease spectrum is very different, and children are more than just 'small adults' when it comes to diagnosis and treatment. In this chapter, we will therefore concentrate on conditions that are specific to children or where there are particular issues relating to the diseases in childhood.

Structural abnormalities of the kidneys and urinary tract

These are commonly detected antenatally (Table 12.1), usually at the 20-week anomaly scan, or in early childhood, often with urinary tract infection (UTI). Some simple examples of congenital urogenital abnormalities are shown in Figure 12.1. Some presentations of UTI are shown in Table 12.2.

Renal pelvic dilatation

This is the most common finding. A fetal renal pelvis of > 5 mm in the anteroposterior diameter is generally considered abnormal,

ABC of Kidney Disease, Second edition.
Edited by David Goldsmith, Satish Jayawardene and Penny Ackland.
© 2013 John Wiley & Sons, Ltd. Published 2013 by John Wiley & Sons, Ltd.

Table 12.1 Antenatal abnormalities of kidneys and urinary tract.

Diagnosis	Features on antenatal scan
Obstruction:	
PUJ	Renal pelvic dilation +/− calyceal dilatation
VUJ	As above, with ureteric dilatation
PUV	As above, with distended bladder; +/−oligohydramnios
Cystic dysplasia	Small, bright, featureless; cysts; +/−oligohydramnios
MCDK	Varying size, non-communicating cysts; no parenchyma
ARPKD	Large, bright, featureless; +/−oligohydramnios
ADPKD	Large, bright; may not see discrete cysts antenatally
Malformation syndromes:	
Bardet−Biedl syndrome	Polydactyly
Meckel−Gruber syndrome	Syndactyly; posterior fossa brain abnormality

ADPKD, autosomal dominant polycystic kidney disease; ARPKD, autosomal recessive polycystic kidney disease; MCDK, multicystic dysplastic kidneys; PUJ, pelvi-ureteric junction, PUV, posterior urethral valve; VUJ, vesico-uretic junction.

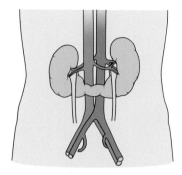

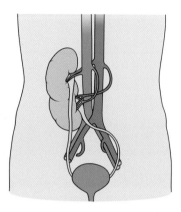

Figure 12.1 Congenital urological abnormalities. (a) Horseshoe kidney. (b) Renal ectopia. (*Source:* Adapted from *Urology*, with permission from Blackwell Publishing Ltd.)

especially if it progresses on serial scans. A common approach is to start prophylactic trimethoprim at birth and perform ultrasound scans at 1 and 6 weeks after birth. If both are normal, then the infant needs no further investigation and prophylaxis can be stopped; 40–50% of postnatal scans will be normal. Severe (> 15 mm) renal pelvic dilatation (RPD), particularly if progressive and associated with intrarenal calyceal dilatation (Figure 12.2), is suggestive of obstruction, either pelviureteric junction obstruction or vesicoureteric junction obstruction if the ureter is also dilated. A Tc-99m MAG-3 (mercaptoacetyltriglycine) renogram will support the diagnosis of obstruction when there is poor drainage, and impaired function on the hydronephrotic side. Surgery (pyeloplasty or ureteric reimplantation) is likely in these cases.

The main area of debate lies in the investigation of infants with mild to moderate (5–15 mm) non-progressive RPD. Common practice includes use of prophylactic trimethoprim for at least the first year, and clinical follow-up with ultrasound monitoring of RPD, but not MCUG (micturating cysto-urethrogram); or an early MCUG and then prophylactic trimethoprim only for infants with proven VUR (vesico-ureteric reflux). In those infants who do

have proven VUR, there is variation in practice over subsequent investigations.

Posterior urethral valve

Posterior urethral valve (PUV) is an important cause of renal failure in male infants and boys. Antenatal RPD is usually bilateral, and associated with ureteric dilatation and a persistently distended bladder. In more severe cases there is cystic change in the renal parenchyma and oligohydramnios, which may lead to pulmonary hypoplasia and life-threatening respiratory failure at delivery. MCUG is essential in this clinical setting (Figure 12.3).

Table 12.2 Presentation of urinary tract infections (UTIs) in children.*

Age group	Most common symptoms	⟶	Least common symptoms
Neonates	Fever, vomiting, lethargy, irritability	Poor feeding, failure to thrive	Abdominal pain, jaundice, haematuria, offensive urine
Preverbal children	Fever	Abdominal pain or abdominal/loin tenderness, vomiting, poor feeding	Lethargy, irritability, haematuria, offensive urine, failure to thrive
Verbal children	Frequent dysuria	Dysfunctional voiding, changes to continence, abdominal pain or tenderness	Fever, malaise, vomiting, haematuria, offensive urine, cloudy urine

*Any child can present with septic shock secondary to UTI, although this is more common in infants. Fever is defined as > 38°C. Children presenting with a UTI need a two-week course of antibiotics and may need referral for imaging to rule out structural abnormalities.

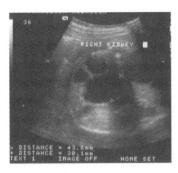

Figure 12.2 Antenatal ultrasound scan showing marked renal pelvic and calyceal dilatation.

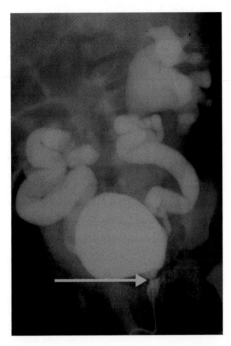

Figure 12.3 Micturating cysto-urethrogram showing filling defect in urethra (PUV) and gross bilateral reflux with dilatation of collecting systems.

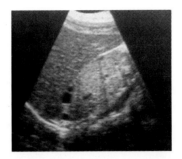

Figure 12.4 Bright featureless dysplastic kidney containing cysts.

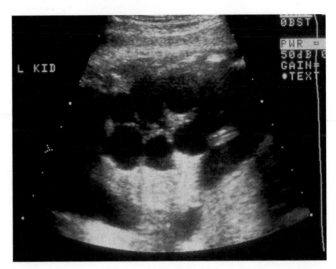

Figure 12.5 Antenatal ultrasound scan showing multiple cysts and absent parenchyma – multicystic dysplastic kidneys.

Meticulous follow-up with combined nephrological and urological care is required. Dialysis and transplantation, and bladder augmentation surgery, may be needed.

Dysplastic kidneys

These are the commonest cause of chronic kidney disease (CKD) overall in infancy and childhood. Antenatal appearances include echobright, featureless and often small kidneys, sometimes with identifiable cysts (Figure 12.4). Oligohydramnios is a sign predicting poor renal function.

Multicystic dysplastic kidneys

Multicystic dysplastic kidneys (MCDK) are usually diagnosed on antenatal scans, and may mimic severe hydronephrosis. There are irregular cysts of variable size from small to several centimetres, and no normal parenchyma (Figure 12.5), with no function on an MAG-3 or DMSA (dimercaptosuccinic) scan. The ureter is

dysplastic and atretic. There is a 20–40% incidence of VUR into the contralateral normal kidney, though if that kidney is normal on ultrasound there is no indication to perform a MCUG. Current practice is not to remove the MCDK unless it is large, increasing in size and causing pressure symptoms.

Duplex kidneys

These are usually detected when one or both moieties are dilated. The commonest abnormalities are:

- obstructed hydronephrotic upper moiety and ureter, often poorly functioning and dysplastic, associated with bladder ureterocoele;
- ectopically inserted upper pole ureter, entering the urethra or vagina; this may cause true continual incontinence with no dry periods at all;
- VUR into lower pole ureter, causing infection and scarring of this pole (Figure 12.6).

Polycystic kidney disease

Polycystic kidney disease in infancy and childhood may be autosomal recessive or dominant. Autosomal recessive polycystic kidney disease (ARPKD) has various clinical presentations, including:

- large echobright kidneys with loss of corticomedullary differentiation on antenatal ultrasound (Figure 12.7);

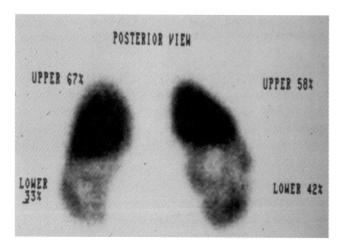

Figure 12.6 Dimercaptosuccinic scan of bilateral duplex kidneys with scarring of both lower moieties.

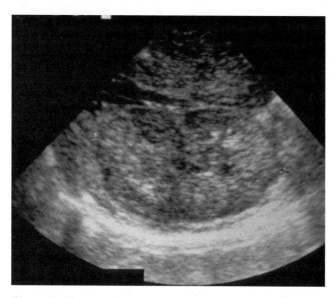

Figure 12.7 Ultrasound showing autosomal recessive polycystic kidney.

- large palpable renal masses and respiratory distress at birth or early infancy;
- signs and symptoms of CKD and hypertension at any time.

The median age for onset of end stage renal failure (ESRF) is around 12 years, though it may cause severe renal failure in infancy; there is very variable disease severity even within the same family. ARPKD is always associated with congenital hepatic fibrosis, which may vary from a subclinical association, to causing liver disease as the dominant clinical feature; complications include ascending cholangitis and portal hypertension.

Inherited, tubular and metabolic diseases

In addition to polycystic kidney disease (above), a number of other genetically determined conditions may present during childhood. The molecular genetic basis is being identified for an increasing number of these conditions.

Alport's syndrome

This is hereditary nephritis with sensorineural deafness and conical deformity of the lens of the eye. It is usually X-linked. Female carriers all have non-visible haematuria, and up to 15% may show some renal impairment in late adult life. It usually presents with an incidental finding of non-visible haematuria, or an episode of visible haematuria. Deafness is first noted around 10 years, hypertension in the mid-teens and it progresses to ESRF at an average age of 21 years.

Nephronophthisis

This is an autosomal recessive condition and the most common genetic cause of ESRF in the first two decades of life. Patients have polyuria from a concentrating defect, giving a history of enuresis and bed-wetting, growth delay, often severe anaemia and a typically 'bland' urinalysis. When associated with tapetoretinal degeneration, it is known as Senior–Løken syndrome.

Bartter's syndrome

This is caused by an autosomal recessive defect leading to profound salt and water wasting. Symptoms are polyuria, polydipsia, episodes of dehydration, failure to thrive and constipation; there may be maternal polyhydramnios. The characteristic biochemical disturbance is hypochloraemic hypokalaemic alkalosis, with inappropriately high levels of urinary Cl^- and Na^+.

Fanconi syndrome

This is characterized by diffuse proximal tubular dysfunction, leading to excess urinary loss of:

- glucose: glycosuria with normal blood glucose;
- phosphate: hypophosphataemic rickets;
- bicarbonate: leading to proximal renal tubular acidosis;
- potassium: causing hypokalaemia;
- sodium, chloride and water: leading to polyuria and polydipsia, chronic extracellular fluid (ECF) volume depletion, failure to thrive and craving for salty foods, e.g. Marmite;
- amino acids: no obvious clinical consequence.

The main causes are rare conditions, including cystinosis, tyrosinaemia, Lowe syndrome (oculocerebrorenal syndrome), galactosaemia, Wilson's disease and heavy metal toxicity (lead, mercury, cadmium).

X-linked hypophosphataemic rickets

This is also known as Vitamin D-resistant rickets, and results in phosphate wasting, hypophosphataemia, delayed growth and rickets. Treatment includes Vitamin D analogues (calcitriol or alfacalcidol) and phosphate supplements. Therapy may be complicated by hypercalcaemia and nephrocalcinosis.

Primary hyperoxaluria

This is an autosomal recessive disorder characterized by an enzyme defect leading to excess hepatic oxalate production and increased urinary excretion, with eventual calcium oxalate precipitation in the kidneys, leading to nephrocalcinosis and renal failure. Therapeutic strategies include isolated liver transplantation, if renal failure has not developed, or combined liver and kidney transplantation.

Idiopathic childhood nephrotic syndrome

Symptoms of adult nephrotic syndrome have been covered in Chapter 7. The incidence of childhood nephrotic syndrome was traditionally quoted as approximately 1 in 50 000 children, until recent information from the United States and elsewhere suggested an increasing incidence (Figure 12.8). Children with steroid-sensitive nephrotic syndrome (80–85% of cases) have a generally good prognosis, although frequently relapsing and steroid-dependent children will need adjunctive treatment. Six months, rather than the conventional course of two months of prednisolone, has been shown to reduce the subsequent frequency of relapse. Alkylating agents, predominantly cyclophosphamide, will induce long-term remissions of up to two years in 50% of children. Levamisole may be useful in a small number of children, and ciclosporin will consistently induce remission, although with the possibility of chronic nephrotoxicity and other adverse events. Mycophenolate mofetil looks to be a promising agent.

Steroid-resistant nephrotic syndrome, usually focal segmental glomerulosclerosis on biopsy, may respond very well to ciclosporin. Unfortunately, recurrent nephrotic syndrome post-transplant occurs in up to 50%, with loss of the graft unless response is seen to intensive immunosuppression with ciclosporin, mycophenonate mofetil (MMF) and plasma exchange.

Glomerulonephritis in children

The commonest form of acute glomerulonephritis (GN) in children is post-streptococcal GN (Box 12.1). With an incidence

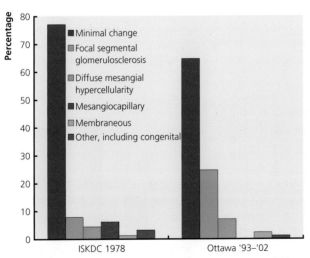

Major published series of cases of nephrotic syndrome in children

Figure 12.8 Changing proportions of children with idiopathic nephrotic syndrome. ISKDC: International Study of Kidney Disease in Children. (*Source:* Reproduced from Filler G *et al.* (2003) Is there really an increase in non-minimal change nephrotic syndrome in children? *Am J Kidney Dis* **42**(6): 1107–13.)

of CKD of 2–5%, mostly in the fulminating cases, it is not always totally benign.

Box 12.1 Glomerulonephritis in children

- Post-streptococcal
- Henoch–Schönlein purpura (HSP)
- Haemolytic uraemic syndrome (HUS)
- IgA nephropathy
- Mesangiocapillary glomerulonephritis
- Vasculitides, e.g.:
  - Systemic lupus erythematosus (SLE)
  - Antineutrophil cytoplasmic antibodies (ANCA) positive vasculitis
- Alport's syndrome
- Membranous nephropathy
- Thin basement membrane disease

Henoch–Schönlein nephritis occurs in 15–62% of children with Henoch–Schönlein purpura (HSP). The majority have a mild, self-limiting course. The risk of progression to ESRF is about 3% of unselected HSP patients, but 25% of those with a severe initial presentation develop renal failure by age 10 years. The outcome in children with IgA nephropathy is similar to that in adults, with about 15% progressing to ESRF.

Chronic vasculitides are occasionally seen, with 10–17% of lupus patients presenting under the age of 16, of whom 50–80% have renal involvement. Children tend to have more severe organ involvement, with a higher mortality (10–20% by age 10 years) and a highly variable five-year kidney survival rate of 44–93%.

Haemolytic uraemic syndrome (HUS) remains the commonest cause (45%) of acute kidney injury (AKI) in childhood. It is usually associated with *E. coli* 0157:H7 enterocolitis, causing severe bloody diarrhoea progressing to AKI and microangiopathic anaemia and thrombocytopenia. The incidence of pneumococcal HUS is increasing in the United Kingdom, Europe and North America. Atypical HUS is exceedingly rare.

Chronic kidney disease

Inherited or congenital conditions account for 50–60% of CKD and ESRF in children. Autosomal recessive diseases are more than twice as common as the cause of ESRF in South Asians compared to the white population (Figures 12.9 and 12.10), and these families require greater input from all aspects of a multidisciplinary service. The aim of management of childhood CKD is to minimize the effects on growth and development, to enable normal (or as near normal as possible) social integration and schooling and to plan for pre-emptive transplantation if appropriate and possible. Key aspects of management of CKD include:

- intensive nutritional support, often with nasogastric or gastrostomy tube feeding;

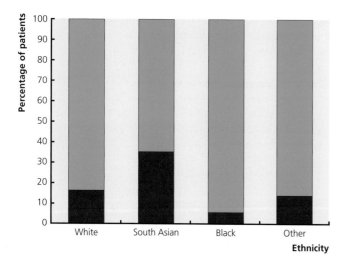

Figure 12.9 Recessive versus other diseases causing end stage renal failure by ethnicity. (*Source*: Renal Registry Data 2006.)

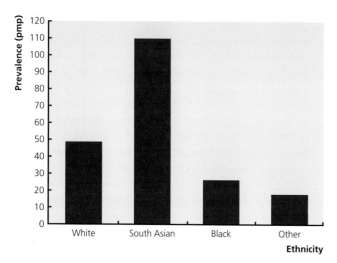

Figure 12.10 Prevalence of end stage renal failure in children by ethnicity. (*Source*: Renal Registry Data 2006.)

- recognition of the need for sodium chloride, sodium bicarbonate and extra fluid supplementation in polyuric dysplastic renal disease (a common cause of CKD);
- management of renal osteodystrophy with dietary phosphate restriction, phosphate binders (usually calcium carbonate) and vitamin D analogues (alfacalcidol);
- use of recombinant human erythropoietin in advanced CKD, to treat anaemia;
- use of recombinant human growth hormone in carefully selected patients.

Infants and children with CKD are often managed by a special clinic with input from a range of professionals including nephrologists, nurse specialists, dieticians and pharmacists.

Renal replacement therapy

In the United Kingdom, the annual average take-on rate for RRT in children < 16 years of age is 7.7/million age-adjusted population,

Table 12.3 Disadvantages of dialysis modalities.

Haemodialysis	Peritoneal
Small vessels, difficult to maintain vascular access	Infection risks, especially infants in nappies or with gastrostomies
Infection risks with long-term tunnelled catheters	May not function if previous abdominal surgery
A-V fistulas associated with impaired arm growth	Parental burnout
Needle phobias and 'wriggly' small children > 3 kg Infants	
Hospital based	
Difficult to maintain education and social interaction	

equating to around 100 patients per year. There are only 13 regional paediatric nephrology centres in the United Kingdom, including one each in Northern Ireland, Wales and Scotland, of which 10 provide transplantation facilities. Dialysis is possible from birth, although, with routine antenatal screening and improved management of labour, it is rarely required so early. Peritoneal dialysis is more practical in very small infants, but is highly stressful for families, with a high rate of 'burnout' (Table 12.3). Dialysis in children is almost always undertaken as an interim treatment with transplantation as the aim. Haemodialysis (HD) is always hospital-based, because of the difficulties maintaining vascular access in small children and their inherent cardiovascular instability. Peritoneal dialysis is usually the modality of choice (Figure 12.11). Care of these children burdens their families with an enormous amount of travelling and disruption to normal family life, with a high rate of marital breakdown and problems with the siblings, who frequently feel ignored and neglected.

Transplantation offers the best quality of life, but, although graft survival rates in children of all ages are now comparable to adults (Table 12.4), regrafting is probably inevitable at some point in the patients' lives. It is thus even more essential to strive towards improved dialysis management and better short- and long-term graft survival in this vulnerable population if we are not merely going to offer adult services to highly sensitized patients with poor

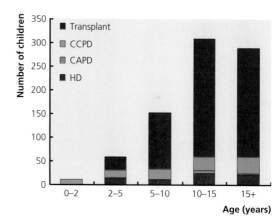

Figure 12.11 Mode of renal replacement therapy with increasing age. CAPD, continuous ambulatory peritoneal dialysis; CCPD, continuous cycling peritoneal dialysis; HD, haemodialysis. (*Source*: Renal Registry Data 2005.)

Table 12.4 Figures from the National Transplant Database for paediatric recipients of first deceased donor and live donor grafts are shown, with comparable adult figures in brackets.

		Number of transplants	Survival estimate (%)
First deceased donor transplants			
One-year survival	Transplant	387 (4991)	90 (88)
	Patient	387 (4991)	99 (95)
Five-year survival	Transplant	434 (5536)	72 (72)
	Patient	434 (5536)	95 (85)
Live donor transplants			
One-year survival	Transplant	189 (1582)	94 (94)
	Patient*	173 (1386)	97 (98)
Five-year survival	Transplant	116 (876)	87 (84)
	Patient*	107 (759)	97 (95)

Survival rates for paediatric (age < 18 years) compared with adult (> 18 years) transplant patients. Cohorts for survival rate estimation: one-year survival, 1 Jan 1999–31 Dec 2003. Five-year survival, 1 Jan 1995–31 Dec 1999. *First grafts only. Regrafts excluded from patient survival estimation.

dialysis access and little hope of retransplantation. Most centres now aim pre-emptively to transplant children in order to avoid dialysis wherever possible, unless medically contraindicated. Paediatric patients receive some priority for deceased donor transplants, but waiting times are increasing, as in the adult sector. Children from ethnic minorities have longer waiting times and lower transplantation rates, as in the adult population. It is technically possible to transplant infants from 10 kg in weight (usually around 2 years in children with CKD), even with an adult kidney, and live donor transplants, usually from a parent, may therefore be considered even at this age. Live donor rates in a few paediatric centres are approaching 75%.

A particularly vulnerable group are adolescents, especially at the time of transfer to adult services, when there is an unacceptably high rate of acute rejection and graft loss due to non-adherence. This is being addressed with the development of more sympathetic and effective transition procedures.

Further reading

Rees L, Webb NJA, Brogan PA (2007) *Paediatric Nephrology (Oxford Specialist Handbooks for Paediatrics)*. Oxford University Press, Oxford.

Webb N, Postlethwaite RJ (eds) (2003) *Clinical Paediatric Nephrology*, 3rd edn. Oxford University Press, Oxford.

CHAPTER 13

The Organization of Services for People with Chronic Kidney Disease: A 21st-Century Challenge

Donal O' Donoghue[1], John Feehally[2] and David Goldsmith[3]

[1]Hope Hospital, Salford, UK
[2]The John Walls Renal Unit, Leicester General Hospital, Leicester, UK
[3]King's College London, London, UK

OVERVIEW

- Around 25% of patients start dialysis without adequate preparation within the United Kingdom. This is often due to a failure to integrate care, such as in patients with diabetes.

- The National Service Framework for kidney disease identifies as markers of best practice in the predialysis phase:
  - multiprofessional care for at least one year before renal replacement therapy (RRT);
  - vascular access at least six months before haemodialysis;
  - pre-emptive transplant listing at a glomerular filtration rate (GFR) of 15 mL/min or six months before dialysis.

- System redesign is required to address the challenges of providing equitable, efficient and high-quality care to people with kidney disease.

- New methods of haemodialysis have emerged. In some units there are patients who are now taking a more independent role in managing their own haemodialysis. 'Home haemodialysis' is also being offered in a growing number of areas. This avoids the travel three times a week to and from the dialysis centre, and the option of overnight dialysis at home allows longer and more efficient sessions.

Introduction

Renal medicine as a clinical speciality is a relative newcomer. Prior to the 1960s, when long-term renal replacement therapy (RRT) first became available as a result of vascular access and transplant surgery, clinical care of people with kidney disease consisted of little more than observing progressive pathophysiology, for which there was little treatment. Care of patients on RRT now provides the major workload for renal teams, although nephrologists still have a significant role in the management of acute kidney injury (AKI) and in the investigation and treatment of a wide range of kidney diseases, which nowadays do not necessarily lead to the need for dialysis.

Until the publication of the Renal National Service Framework (NSF) policy in the United Kingdom in 2004/5, initiatives focused

exclusively on dialysis and transplantation. It is now recognized that the renal care pathway is much broader. A preventative dividend may be achieved if we had a better understanding of factors responsible for the initiation of renal injury and by the early detection and active management of progressive kidney disease.

There is now a clear appreciation of by how much the numbers of people affected by some degree of chronic kidney disease (CKD) are increasing (Box 13.1). This has been labelled an 'epidemic' in some quarters. This large expansion in affected individuals has been fuelled both by global increases in obesity and type 2 diabetes mellitus (Figure A4.1, Appendix 4) and by a better understanding of how to describe the earlier manifestations of CKD – in terms of microalbuminuria, and early reduction in renal function (GFR) (Box 13.2).

Box 13.1 **Key facts**

Chronic kidney disease

- >5% of population
- comorbidity: 90% HT, 40% CVD, 20% DM
- SMR 36 in unreferred <60 years
- optimal therapy 30%
- potential savings in United States $18–60 bn/10 years

End stage renal failure

- increased at 6–8% p.a.; until mid-2000s – now static in many countries
- acute uraemic emergencies 25%, (see Appendix 4, Figure A4.2)
- pre-emptive transplant listing 3–54%
- dialysis survival 1st year 85–95%
- cost £0.4 bn/year (2002/03) rising to >£0.8 bn/year (2010/11).

HT, hypertension; CVD, cardiovascular disease; DM, diabetes mellitus; SMR, standard mortality rate

---

The 2007 model of service

Services for people with kidney disease in the United Kingdom originally developed in teaching hospitals, mostly alongside academic departments, but have over the last 30 years expanded into some district hospitals. Over that time the number of people on RRT has

ABC of Kidney Disease, Second edition.
Edited by David Goldsmith, Satish Jayawardene and Penny Ackland.
© 2013 John Wiley & Sons, Ltd. Published 2013 by John Wiley & Sons, Ltd.

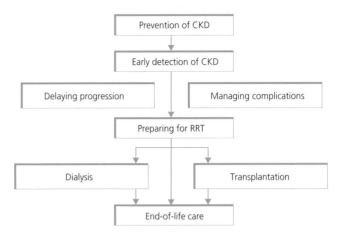

Figure 13.1 The kidney patient pathway.

a central pillar of the Renal NSF, requires information systems that work across institutional, professional and geographic barriers. This can be achieved, but current realization is patchy across the United Kingdom and will require sustained investment and resources.

Box 13.3 **The challenges facing renal health care**

- Integrating CKD management into other vascular disease programmes
- Expansion of dialysis services
- Increasing the number of kidney donors
- Establishing supportive and palliative care for people with CKD

more than quadrupled. Yet by international comparison, the United Kingdom lagged significantly behind other developed countries in the provision of renal services, especially France and Germany. The renal community of care remains small, with only 80 main renal departments providing in-patient services. Twenty-three of these are combined with a transplant unit on-site. In the last decade, outreach clinics have been established in many district hospitals. Satellite units providing dialysis for stable patients are now much more numerous, and more than half of all haemodialysis patients are now managed in these local units. Despite this growth, for the majority of patients the travelling time for haemodialysis, which is a thrice-weekly treatment, remains in excess of the standard of less than 30 minutes.

One of the major continuing challenges is the development of new renal services alongside the continued necessary expansion of existing dialysis and renal units. Changes in patterns of working to achieve this are both inevitable and increasingly desirable. Renal services need a stable commissioning and planning platform from which to respond to local needs.

Challenges for renal health care

The 'historical' centralized model of care is ill-equipped to manage the epidemic of CKD and provide long-term support across the whole kidney patient pathway, much of which by definition will take place in a community setting (Figure 13.1). System redesign was required to address the challenges of providing equitable, timely, efficient and high-quality care to people with kidney disease (Box 13.3). Although the number of consultant nephrologists has almost doubled in the last 10 years, and this growth continues, albeit slowly, investment in education and training of the whole renal multiprofessional team is required to provide a motivated, flexible and empowered workforce to meet the needs of these patients. Of greatest importance is the understanding that community-based or primary care must play an increasingly important role in this endeavour, complementing other groups. An integrated care plan,

The roles of primary care

Inclusion of a CKD domain within the Quality and Outcomes Framework (QOF) of the General Medical Services (GMS) Contract from April 2006 has placed the emphasis for the detection of early kidney disease in primary care (Table 13.1). Establishing practice-based registers of CKD is the cornerstone of chronic disease management. The universal adoption in 2006 of the KDOQI (Kidney Dialysis Outcomes Quality Initiative) classification of the stages of CKD and the automatic reporting of estimated glomerular filtration rates (eGFR) by clinical chemistry laboratories now

Table 13.1 The chronic kidney disease domain of Quality and Outcomes Framework (2006/7).

	Points	Payment stages
CKD1: A register of patients aged 18 years and over with CKD (stage 3–5 CKD)	6	
CKD2: Percentage of patients with a record of BP in the last 15 months	6	40–90%
CKD3: Percentage of patients with a BP of 140/85 or less	11	40–70%
CKD4: Percentage of patients who are treated with an ACEI and ARB (unless a contraindication)	4	40–80%

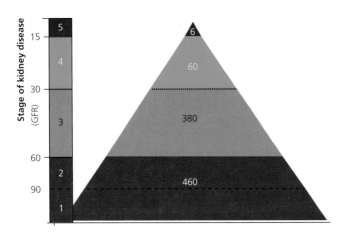

Figure 13.2 Chronic kidney disease in a typical GP practice of 10 000.

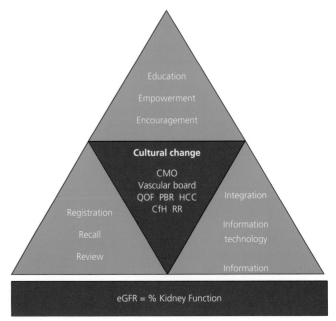

Figure 13.3 Demystifying and managing chronic renal disease. CfH, Connecting for Health; CMO, chief medical officer; HCC, Health Care Commission; PBR, payment by results; QOF, Quality and Outcomes Framework, RR, Renal Registry.

facilitate the creation of these registers. Those at risk of CKD have been defined by the Renal NSF. See Figure 13.2 for the situation in the average GP practice. From community-based research, we know that the majority of those with moderate to severe CKD are already having serial serum creatinine measurements. Some of these are opportunistic, often during an intercurrent illness, while others are part of regular monitoring of people known to have hypertension, vascular disease or diabetes.

Recall of those on the *register* for *regular review*, the three Rs of chronic disease management, will enable a systematic approach to patient management to be implemented. The importance of vascular risk reduction in improving vascular and renal outcomes has already been emphasized in previous chapters.

There is an opportunity to integrate vascular care using the same GP-based systems for coronary heart disease, kidney disease, diabetes and stroke (Figure A4.3). However, the perception that kidney disease is complex, rare and always requires specialist care is inimical to such a holistic approach. Demystifying kidney disease and its management (one of the aims of this book) requires a shift in the paradigm from serum creatinine to eGFR, alongside the use of 'percentage kidney function' as the currency of kidney disease in the education of healthcare professionals and particularly in the empowerment of people with kidney disease (Figure 13.3).

For the majority of those with kidney disease, an appreciation of their increased vascular risk, especially with diabetes, and inclusion of interventions to minimize this in their care plan, is required. A minority where the diagnosis is unclear, with features of progression (such as proteinuria, falling eGFR or uncontrolled hypertension) or with the complications of advanced CKD, can benefit most from specialist care.

The recently published UK guidelines on the management of CKD (NICE 2008) provide referral templates. We know from the falling rates of coronary heart disease and cancer in many parts of the world that such a population-based systematic approach to care can be effective.

Planning for renal replacement therapy

Patients who arrive as 'crash-landers' (with advanced CKD, but unknown to local renal services [Figure A4.2]) requiring urgent unplanned dialysis have poorer outcomes compared to those who have experienced educational programmes, been given the opportunity to make informed choices regarding RRT modality and start dialysis in a planned fashion or receive a pre-emptive transplant (see Chapters 9–11). These 'crash' patients have twice the mortality and three times the length of hospitalization in their first year on dialysis. In the United Kingdom, depending on where patients live around 25%, of people start dialysis without this adequate preparation. In many cases, such as in people with diabetes, this almost certainly reflects a failure to integrate care. The Renal NSF identifies multiprofessional care for at least one year, vascular access surgery six months before haemodialysis and pre-emptive transplant listing at a GFR of 15 mL/min or six months before dialysis, as markers of best practice in the predialysis phase (Box 13.4).

Box 13.4 Predialysis care: NSF markers of good practice

- Referral to a multiskilled team, if possible at least one year before start of dialysis
- Accelerated, intensive input from renal team for those who present late
- People with ESRF given information about all forms of treatment so that informed choice can be made
- Patients put on transplant list within six months of their anticipated start of dialysis
- Anaemia treated to maintain an adequate haemoglobin level
- Management of cardiovascular risk factors and diabetes according to NSFs for coronary heart disease and diabetes

(See Chapters 3, 5, 9, 10, 11)

Predialysis services are underdeveloped. A recent survey found that an estimated number of 140 000 CKD patients were under the care of UK nephrologists but few units had access to the full complement of the recommended multiskilled team. Counsellors and psychologists were the most commonly perceived shortages, and the current provision of service was found to be patchy and variable.

Dialysis and transplantation

RRT requires additional skills to predialysis care. This includes catering for critically ill people with AKI, those requiring intense immunosuppression and those with complex metabolic disarray. In contrast to predialysis care, however, we have high-quality activity and performance data for long-term dialysis and renal transplantation from the UK Renal Registry and UK Transplant. The UK Renal Registry has achieved universal coverage for all patients on RRT in the United Kingdom and has long-established robust audit arrangements that provide an ideal vehicle for continual quality improvement of care. The challenge here is to ensure that the development of Connecting for Health builds on this expertise and provides additional functionality to extend the scope of comparative national audit.

The delivery of patient-centred care has always been a challenge which renal medicine has relished; renal units have many long-standing 'expert' patients who rightly understand the importance of excellent information and proper communication to assist their decision-making. This has now been taken one step further with Renal Patient View, a unique system developed by the renal community that allows patients direct personal Web-based access to appropriate information directly downloaded from clinical information systems in renal units.

Transplantation is the best form of RRT for those that are suitable – which is up to 40% of those receiving dialysis. Figure 13.4 shows that for the first time in many years transplantation now represents less than 50% of the total population receiving RRT. Transplantation, particularly live donation, has unique challenges, which include paying attention to societal views, increasing public awareness and garnering support. Transplantation care is much wider than the kidney engraftment operation itself, and the periods immediately before and after this. It includes recipient preparation, donor care, relationships with critical care colleagues and long-term post-transplant care with its elements of increased vascular risk, complications of CKD and unusual pattern of malignancy risks.

Independent sector treatment centres

One aspect of renal care – the maintenance of thrice-weekly outpatient haemodialysis – is potentially suitable for a differing model of healthcare delivery, such as the independent sector treatment centres (ISTCs), which are now being vigorously adopted. The concept is not new to renal care. There is a 30-year experience in this country of offering maintenance dialysis in satellite dialysis facilities built and maintained by (private) specialist dialysis companies. Many of the issues that concern observers of the ISTC innovation – including achieving proper quality control, ensuring seamless transition between the independent sector and the NHS when required, proper information transfer and uniform standards of care – have all long been resolved by NHS renal units working with their commercial partners in such facilities. Experience dictates that with open tendering private providers sometimes, but not always, win contracts for such satellite units and can offer significant value for money.

Supportive and palliative care in chronic kidney disease

CKD is a disease of older people and is associated with a range of comorbidities (Box 13.5). Many patients elect not to have dialysis as their long-term prognosis and quality of life independent of CKD are poor. This important area is explored more fully in Chapter 9.

Box 13.5 **Criteria for supportive care in CKD**

At least two of the indicators below

- CKD stage 5 (eGFR < 15 mL/min)
- Frail individuals at CKD stage 4 (eGFR 15–25 mL/min)
- Patients thought to be in the last year of life by the care team: the 'surprise question'
- Patients choosing the no dialysis option, discontinuing dialysis or opting not to restart dialysis if their transplant is failing
- Difficult physical symptoms (e.g. anorexia, nausea, pruritus, reduced function status, intractable fluid overload) or psychological symptoms despite optimal tolerated therapy

---

Current developments (See Appendix 4)

Over recent years there has been much good progress in the UK. This has occurred by sound investment, and leveraging primary care performance in terms of earlier detection of CKD and appropriate early interventions, for example, when albuminuria is detected on screening. Our dialysis "take-on" rates are almost certainly appropriate at last. The gap between ourselves and other industrialised countries is narrowing (Ansell, 2010). There has been a significant and welcomed expansion in renal pallation; indeed, most renal

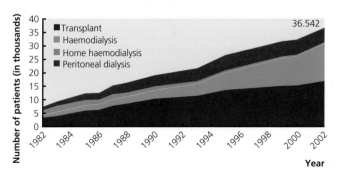

Figure 13.4 Renal replacement therapy modalities.

units would now be able to offer a good service. Choice of dialysis modality is a real option for the majority of patients; it should be something we strive to offer all. In particular, there is growth, still patchy in places, in home dialysis provision, with many units considering peritoneal and home haemodialysis as complementary to one another as "home dialysis therapies". Pre-emptive and living donor/altruistic kidney transplantation has also grown significantly, as has our ability to manage more complex immunological challenges. All of this is good and encouraging. There is of course very much more work to do. Especially if one has as the goal to eliminate unwanted variation in delivery and patient experience of healthcare. Of course, some variation is to be celebrated, especially if this represents innovation and fresh thinking.

On a broader global setting, this pattern in advanced industrialised countries has been mirrored. The big challenge now, with the global economical strains so evident, is to continue to provide more, provide it faster and more responsively, while staying cost neutral. This will require ever more ingenious and flexible ways of working to be embraced and encouraged. In the developing world, by contrast, there remain startling inequities of access to renal replacement therapy which in many countries remains far from a basic healthcare right. The big challenges here are around the fact that in 2012 and beyond, non-communicable diseases now kill more people in say Africa than the old traditional killers of infections such as TB, Leprosy, Malaria and HIV. Healthcare systems are thus doubly challenged by old killers and new ones making invidious spending/investment choices inevitable.

Prevention of renal disease (earlier detection and intervention) have to be the priority for countries which often cannot begin to afford the complex healthcare infrastructure we sometimes take for granted in industrialised countries.

Conclusion

CKD is a long-term condition, whose frequency is increasing. Provision of dialysis facilities is very expensive. Prevention makes huge societal, medical and financial sense. Part of CKD care will occur in an acute setting, and hospitals are likely to remain the major provider of RRT programmes. But to achieve the integrated care necessary for an efficient, high-quality service envisioned by the Renal NSF, commissioning of pathways of care will be necessary so that resources can be made available at the right part of the pathway at the right time.

References

Ansell, D, Risdale, S and Caskey, F (2010) Changing patterns of renal replacement therapy. In *Supportive Care of the Renal Patient*, 2nd edition. Oxford University Press, Oxford. www.books.google.co.uk/books?isbn =019956003X.

NICE (2008) Clinical Guideline 73: Chronic kidney disease, http://www .nice.org.uk/CG073.

Further reading

NSF Parts 1 and 2, http://www.dh.gov.uk/PolicyAndGuidance/HealthAnd SocialCareTopics/Renal/fs/en.

Renal Registry and Renal Registry Report, http://www.renalreg.com.

The Renal Association, http://www.renal.org/ and http://www.renal.org/ eGFR/eguide.html.

UK Transplant, http://www.uktransplant.org.uk.

Chronic Kidney Disease and Drug Prescribing

Douglas Maclean[†1], Satish Jayawardene[2] and Hayley Wells[1]

[1]Guy's and St Thomas' NHS Foundation Trust, London, UK
[2]King's College Hospital NHS Foundation Trust, London, UK

Many commonly prescribed medicines are metabolized or excreted by the kidney. Impaired renal function can alter drug behaviour in the body, including:

- reduction in renal excretion of a drug or its metabolites may lead to potential accumulation and associated toxic effects;
- the build-up of uraemic toxins may be associated with alterations in behaviour of drugs within the body;
- alterations in absorption of medicines, e.g. reduction in the absorption of furosemide following oral administration in patients with visceral oedema;
- changes in sensitivity of the body to some drugs even if elimination is not compromised, e.g. opiates increase cerebral sensitivity;
- tissue distribution of certain drugs may alter as a consequence of accumulation of body water and/or reduced renal clearance of uraemic toxins, e.g. antibiotics including gentamicin, amikacin;
- binding of drugs to proteins in the blood may be reduced in nephrotic syndrome, e.g. flucloxacillin, phenytoin and sodium valproate, with increased risk of toxicity.

Many of these factors have implications for drug prescribing in patients with compromised renal function, in terms of the choice of drug and the dose prescribed. Failure to consider these may place such patients at increased risk of drug-related adverse effects, including renal toxicity.

Dosing regimens based on glomerular filtration (mainly creatinine clearance estimates) should be used when administering drugs with a narrow therapeutic window, e.g. anti-arrhythmics such as *disopyramide, flecainide, nadolol, sotalol,* in addition to other agents, including *aciclovir, gabapentin, digoxin, ethambutol, lithium* and *methotrexate.* For many of these drugs, whose efficacy and toxicity are closely related to serum concentrations, dosing should be determined both in terms of clinical response and quantifiable measures, e.g. international normalized ratio (INR) for patients undergoing treatment with warfarin. Serum levels can also be useful to aid drug dosing, allowing optimization of clinical effect with minimization of toxicity. See also Table A1.1.

[†]Deceased.

ABC of Kidney Disease, Second edition.
Edited by David Goldsmith, Satish Jayawardene and Penny Ackland.
© 2013 John Wiley & Sons, Ltd. Published 2013 by John Wiley & Sons, Ltd.

Drugs that may impair kidney function

Drugs can be nephrotoxic through a variety of pathophysiological mechanisms, including pre-renal hypoperfusion (e.g. captopril), glomerulopathy (e.g. penicillamine, gold), allergic interstitial nephritis (e.g. antibiotics, proton pump inhibitors), direct tubular toxicity (e.g. aminoglycosides, high-dose rosuvastatin) and tubular obstruction (e.g. sulphonamides). Patient factors such as dehydration, sepsis, pre-existing heart failure and concomitant drug therapy (e.g. nonsteroidal anti-inflammatory drugs, or NSAIDs, diuretics and ACE inhibitors/angiotensin II receptor blockers) will increase inherent risk of drug-related toxicity.

Drugs affected by pre-existing kidney disease

The renal excretion of many drugs may depend on the glomerular filtration rate (GFR), a balance between secretion and reabsorption of drugs in the renal tubules or renal drug metabolism, e.g. insulin and interferons. When GFR is reduced in renal disease, the clearance of drugs eliminated by the kidney is decreased and the plasma half-life is prolonged, e.g. aciclovir, opiates, digoxin and sotalol.

Drug prescribing in renal impairment

Special care is required when interpreting advice on dose adjustment based on creatinine clearance (e.g. calculated from the Cockcroft and Gault formula) because renal function is increasingly being reported on the basis of estimated glomerular filtration rate (eGFR) normalized to a body surface area of $1.73 \, m^2$ and derived from the MDRD (Modification of Diet in Renal Disease) formula. **The two measures of renal function cannot be used interchangeably.**

Pain management in patients with chronic kidney disease

Pain is one of the most common symptoms experienced by patients with chronic kidney disease (CKD); it impairs their quality of life and is undertreated.

The World Health Organization (WHO) three-step analgesic ladder is a helpful aid to guidance on pain management in these patients (Figure A1.1).

Paracetamol 500 mg to 1 g four times a day given regularly should be considered for mild pain associated with CKD. Paracetamol is

Table A1.1 Commonly prescribed anti-infective drugs in adults with pre-existing chronic kidney disease. Seek expert advice for patients undergoing dialysis.

Drug	Creatinine clearance (mL/min/1.73 m²)	Dosage
Aciclovir oral Herpes Zoster:	>25 mL/min	800 mg five times a day
	10–25 mL/min	800 mg every 8 hours
	<10 mL/min	800 mg every 12 hours
Aciclovir oral Herpes Simplex:	>25 mL/min	200 mg five times a day or 400 mg five times a day in immunosuppressed patients
	10–25 mL/min	Dose 3–4 times a day
	<10 mL/min	Dose every 12 hours
Aciclovir iv	>50 mL/min	5–10 mg/kg (depending on indication) every 8 hours. Dose using ideal body weight
	<50 mL/min	See local guidelines and seek expert advice
Amoxicillin		250–500 mg every 8 hours. No dose adjustment required in renal impairment
Benzylpenicillin iv	>125 mL/min	2.4–14.4 g (depending on indication) daily in 4–6 divided doses
	<125 mL/min	See local guidelines and seek expert advice
Cefaclor		250 mg every 8 hours. No dose adjustment required in renal impairment
Cefadroxil	>50 mL/min	1 g every 12–24 hours
	25–50 mL/min	500–1000 mg every 12 hours
	10–25 mL/min	500–1000 mg every 24 hours
	<10 mL/min	500–1000 mg every 36 hours
Cefuroxime iv	>20 mL/min	750–1.5 g every 8 hours
	10–20 mL/min	750 mg every 12 hours
	<10 mL/min	750 mg every 24 hours
Ceftazidime iv	>50 mL/min	0.5–2 g every 8–12 hours
	31–50 mL/min	1–2 g every 12 hours
	16–30 mL/min	1–2 g every 24 hours
	6–15 mL/min	500 mg–1 g every 24 hours
	<5 mL/min	500 mg–1 g every 48 hours
Cefalexin	>20 mL/min	250 mg every 6 hours or 500 mg every 8–12 hours. Recurrent UTI prophylaxis: 125 mg every night
	10–20 mL/min	500 mg every 8–12 hours
	<10 mL/min	250–500 mg every 8–12 hours
Cefradine	>10 mL/min	250–500 mg every 6 hours or 500 mg–1 g every 12 hours
	<10 mL/min	250–500 mg every 6 hours
Ciprofloxacin oral	>60 mL/min	250–750 mg every 12 hours
	30–60 mL/min	250–500 mg every 12 hours
	<30 mL/min	250 mg–500 mg every 24 hours
Ciprofloxacin iv	>60 mL/min	100–400 mg every 12 hours
	30–60 mL/min	200–400 mg every 12 hours
	<30 mL/min	200–400 mg every 24 hours
Clindamycin	>10 mL/min	150–450 mg every six hours
	<10 mL/min	Half-life increased consider reducing dose
Clarithromycin	>30 mL/min	250–500 mg every 12 hours
	<30 mL/min	250 mg every 12 hours
Co-amoxiclav oral	>30 mL/min	375–625 mg every 8 hours
	10–30 mL/min	375–625 mg every 12 hours
	<10 mL/min	375–625 mg every 24 hours
Co-amoxiclav iv	>30 mL/min	1.2 g every 8 hours
	10–30 mL/min	Initial 1.2 g and then 600 mg given every 12 hours
	<10 mL/min	Initial 1.2 g and then 600 mg given every 24 hours
Co-trimoxazole	>30 mL/min	960 mg every 12 hours. PCP 120 mg/kg/day in 2–4 divided doses
	<30 mL/min	Seek expert advice
Doxycycline		Normal dose 50–200 mg every 24 hours depending on indication. No dose adjustment required in renal impairment
Erythromycin	>10 mL/min	250–500 mg every 6 hours or 500 mg–1 g every 12 hours
	<10 mL/min	Maximum total daily dose <1.5 g
Flucloxacillin	>10 mL/min	250–500 mg every 6 hours (higher doses in endocarditis)
	<10 mL/min	No dose adjustment required in renal impairment Up to a max 4 g/day
Fluconazole	>50 mL/min	50–400 mg every 24 hours
	<50 mL/min	No adjustments in single dose therapy are required. Reduce to 50% of dose

Table A1.1 (continued)

Drug	Creatinine clearance (mL/min/1.73 m^2)	Dosage
Gentamicin iv		See local guidelines and seek expert advice.
Meropenem iv	>50 mL/min 26–50 mL/min 10–25 mL/min <10 mL/min	500 mg–2 g every 8 hours Dose every 12 hours 50% of dose every 12 hours 50% of dose every 24 hours
Metronidazole		Orally 200–400 mg every 8 hours IV 500 mg every 8 hours. No dose adjustment required in renal impairment
Nitrofurantoin	>60 mL/min <60 mL/min	50–100 mg every 6 hours Contraindicated as adequate urinary concentrations are not achieved
Ofloxacin	>50 mL/min 20–50 mL/min <20 mL/min	200–400 mg every 24 hours Normal loading dose, then reduce to 50% every 24 hours Normal loading dose, 100 mg should be given every 24 hours
Terbinafine	>50 mL/min <50 mL/min	250 mg every 24 hours 250 mg every 48 hours
Tetracycline	>10 mL/min <10 mL/min	250–500 mg every 6 hours 250 mg every 6 hours. Caution: will artificially increase serum creatinine
Trimethoprim	>25 mL/min <25 mL/min	200 mg every 12 hours Dose as in normal renal function for 1 day then 100 mg every 12 hours. Caution: will artificially increase serum creatinine
Vancomycin iv	>50 mL/min <50 mL/min	1 g every 12 hours See local guidelines and seek expert advice

available in various dose formulations, including liquid, tablets and soluble tablets and suppositories. No dosage modification is required for any degree of impaired renal function.

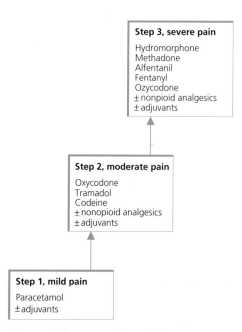

Step 3, severe pain

Hydromorphone
Methadone
Alfentanil
Fentanyl
Ozycodone
±nonpioid analgesics
±adjuvants

Step 2, moderate pain

Oxycodone
Tramadol
Codeine
±nonpioid analgesics
±adjuvants

Step 1, mild pain

Paracetamol
±adjuvants

Figure A1.1 The WHO three-step analgesic ladder. Adjuvant analgesics are added to enhance analgesia such as steroids for pain from bone metastases. Adjuvants also include medication such as anticonvulsants for neuropathic pain, e.g. gabapentin, pregabalin and antidepressants, e.g. amitriptyline, fluoxetine. (*Source:* Adapted from Barakzoy AS and Moss AH (2006) Efficacy of the World Health Organization analgesic ladder to treat pain in end-stage renal disease. *J Am Soc Nephrolo* **17**: 3198–203.)

Nonsteroidal anti-inflammatory drugs

All NSAIDs should be avoided in patients with mild to moderate impaired renal function. They can further dramatically accelerate the rate of decline of renal function. Patients may also be predisposed to uraemic gastritis and gastrointestinal (GI) bleeding.

Cyclooxygenase inhibitors (COX-1) include diclofenac, ibuprofen, mefenamic acid, naproxen, indomethacin and sulindac (a pro-drug that must be converted into its active form by the kidneys).

COX-2 inhibitors such as celecoxib and meloxicam, although believed to cause fewer adverse GI effects, should be prescribed with caution in these patients.

In end stage renal failure, nonsteroidal drugs can be prescribed for patients where the clinical benefits outweigh the risks, usually in conjunction with gastroprotectant agents such as H2 receptor antagonists, e.g. ranitidine, or non-renally cleared proton pump inhibitors, including omeprazole.

Other analgesic options are shown in Table A1.2.

Parenteral diamorphine or morphine, especially if intravenous, should be administered with extreme caution in patients with compromised renal function, as active metabolites that are renally excreted can accumulate. Diamorphine and morphine should only be prescribed when the therapeutic benefits clearly outweigh the clinical risks. It should be borne in mind that intravenous, intramuscular and subcutaneous doses of either diamorphine or morphine are not equipotent in terms of analgesic potency. If either of these drugs is to be administered, it should be commenced at the lowest doses available and reviewed regularly.

Table A1.2 Other analgesic options.

Drug	Normal Dose Range	Modified dosing range for compromised renal function (creatinine clearance: mL/min)
Codeine phosphate	30 mg 4-hourly	>10 mL/min dose as in normal renal function Less than 10 mL/min increase dosing interval to 6-hourly
Tramadol	Oral 50–100 mg at intervals of not less than 4 hours	Greater than 30 mL/min dose as in normal renal function 10–30 mL/min, normal dose every 12 hours Less than 10 mL/min 50 mg every 12 hours
Oxycodone	5 mg every 4–6 hours to a maximum daily dose of 400 mg Modified release capsules can be administered initially at a dose of 10 mg every 12 hours titrating gradually	Start initially at 2.5 mg every 8–12 hours and titrate slowly according to individual patient's response
Fentanyl	50–200 µg by subcutaneous injection then 50 µg as required Topical formulations of fentanyl include lozenges and transdermal patches. Specialist advice should be sought for its use	10–20 mL/min, 75% of normal dose Less than 10 mL/min, 50% of normal, titrate according to individual patient's response

Table A1.3 Commonly prescribed drugs.

Drug	Usual dose	Notes
Sodium bicarbonate	500 mg–2 g three times a day	Used to treat the acidosis of renal failure Also helps lower serum potassium levels
ACEI/ARB	Depending upon formulation used	Used to reduce blood pressure and proteinuria Essential to check renal function and potassium 10–14 days following initiation
Calcium-based phosphate binders (calcium carbonate or calcium acetate)	Depending upon formulation used	Taken with meals to bind phosphate Dose adjusted according to phosphate and calcium levels
Non-calcium-based phosphate binders (sevelamer or aluminium hydroxide)	Depending upon formulation used	Taken with meals to bind phosphate Dose adjusted according to phosphate levels Used in those who are hypercalcaemic
Iron (as various formulations for IV use)	200–500 mg (posology depending on manufacturer's instructions, haemoglobin, serum ferritin, and other indices of iron status; see Chapter 5)	Given to anaemic patients who are iron-deficient
ESAs (e.g. darbepoetin alfa, epoetin alfa, epoetin beta, methoxy polyethylene glycol-epoetin beta)	Dose and frequency depends upon formulation and haemoglobin level	For management of anaemia associated with renal impairment
Alfacalcidol	Usually 0.25–1 µg once daily	Is a vitamin D analogue For the treatment of secondary hyperparathyroidism
N-acetyl cysteine	600 mg twice daily (4 doses)	Used for the prevention of contrast nephrotoxicity

ACEI, angiotensin converting enzyme inhibitor; ARB, angiotensin II receptor blocker; ESAs, Erythropoietin stimulating agents.

Prescribing for patients with chronic kidney disease/end stage renal failure

Table A1.3 shows a list of drugs that are commonly prescribed in those patients with CKD. They are used especially in those with stages 3, 4 and 5 kidney disease. They are used to treat the symptoms and clinical sequelae of CKD/end stage renal failure.

Further resources

Ashley C, Currie A (eds) (2009) *The Renal Drug Handbook*, 3nd edn. Radcliffe Medical Press, Oxford.

Barakzoy AS, Moss AH (2006) Efficacy of the World Health Organization Analgesic Ladder to treat pain in end-stage renal disease. *J Am Soc Nephrol* **17**: 3198–203.

Mehta, D (ed.) (2011) *British National Formulary 62*. Pharmaceutical Press, London.

APPENDIX 2

Glossary of Renal Terms and Conditions

David Goldsmith

King's College London, London, UK

This section provides a quick reference guide for those 'diagnoses' that so often appear in discharge summaries from renal teams to GPs and other non-nephrology consultants. We provide only the bare bones of a description and the key things to know. Anyone interested in more detailed learning can use one or more of the many online resources to which we have provided links.

Alport's syndrome

See Chapter 12.

Anti-GBM (Goodpasture's) disease

This is a very rare disease that is a small vessel vasculitis involving the renal capillaries (presenting as acute kidney injury (AKI)/rapidly progressive glomerulonephritis, or RPGN) and sometimes the pulmonary capillaries (presenting as acute severe pulmonary haemorrhage).

Diagnosis is made on clinical grounds, and backed up by changes in chest X-ray, lung function testing, circulating anti-GBM antibodies (performed by specialized immunology laboratories) and renal biopsy.

Typically, this is an aggressive one-shot illness seen in younger patients, and results in rapid renal failure or fatal lung bleeding. Aggressive immunosuppression including plasma exchange can reduce the risk from lung haemorrhage, but rarely can severe/permanent renal failure be prevented.

Autosomal dominant polycystic kidney disease

See Chapter 6.

Diabetic nephropathy (DN)

Diabetes (type 1 and 2) constitutes the commonest current cause of end stage renal failure (ESRF) in the industrialized world. Type 2 diabetes is rapidly increasing in prevalence and, although often a disease of middle to old age, is occurring more frequently in younger age groups as global obesity increases.

In about a third of patients, renal involvement can occur, usually after 10–20 years of diabetes (diabetic nephropathy is a small vessel complication, such as sensorimotor/autonomic neuropathy, retinopathy and small arteriolar disease). The first sign of renal involvement by diabetic nephropathy is microalbuminuria (MAU) (see Chapter 1). Early treatment with angiotensin converting enzyme inhibitors (ACEIs) and angiotensin receptor blockers (ARBs), to lower blood pressure (BP) and reduce MAU, can abort the otherwise inevitable progression to overt proteinuria and renal functional decline.

It is of the greatest importance that all patients with diabetes have annual urine testing for the presence of MAU, and have meticulous attention paid to overall metabolic control, dyslipidaemia and BP. Cardiovascular disease is very common in all diabetics, the more so in those with any degree of renal disease.

Focal segmental glomerulosclerosis

Focal segmental glomerulosclerosis (FSGS) is a diagnostic term for a clinicopathological syndrome with multiple aetiologies. FSGS is becoming a more common renal condition, and is the commonest renal lesion (excepting diabetic nephropathy) in black patients. It can be idiopathic, or secondary to other renal pathologies and lesions.

Presentation can be at any age, and is usually with isolated proteinuria or more commonly nephrotic syndrome. Hypertension and renal impairment are common.

Diagnosis is by means of renal biopsy. Treatment can be effected by ACEI and ARBs to reduce proteinuria and BP. Long courses of prednisolone, or other immunosuppressants, can help in selected cases.

Glomerulonephritis

Glomerulonephritis (GN; see Chapter 12, p. 75) covers glomerular disease, is often (but not always) inflammatory in nature and can be primary or secondary to another systemic illness (e.g. lupus).

GN causes raised BP, oedema, renal impairment, non-visible haematuria (sometimes visible) and significant proteinuria

ABC of Kidney Disease, Second edition.
Edited by David Goldsmith, Satish Jayawardene and Penny Ackland.
© 2013 John Wiley & Sons, Ltd. Published 2013 by John Wiley & Sons, Ltd.

(PCR > 100). There may also be signs relating to any underlying inflammatory, degenerative, metabolic or other systemic processes (e.g. vasculitic rash).

Depending on the type of GN, the age of the patient and the extent of reversible versus irreversible renal damage, there can be therapies to retard or regress the GN. Acute renal vasculitis can be effectively treated with potent immunosuppressives.

IgA disease and Henoch–Schönlein purpura

IgA-nephropathy (IgA-N) is a form of primary GN, and is the commonest form of primary GN in most parts of the world. It occurs in all age groups, but is most common in younger people (children and adolescents). In younger patients, recurrent visible haematuria, and intermittent or persistent proteinuria, with hypertension, are the commonest presentations. Exacerbations of symptoms often occur with febrile illnesses, or upper respiratory tract infection/tonsillitis. In older subjects, the signs are less dramatic as visible haematuria is rarer. IgA-N is a significant cause of isolated non-visible haematuria (see Chapter 1).

Particularly in children and adolescents, but more rarely in adults, there can be a symptom complex of vasculitic rash on extensor surfaces, arthralgia, gastrointestinal pain and haemorrhage (e.g. rectal bleeding) with acute IgA-N. This is known as Henoch–Schönlein purpura (HSP). Antipyretics, analgesics and sometimes steroids can help the systemic features.

The diagnosis can only be made by renal biopsy, and this is essential as other forms of glomerular disease can present in similar ways. Treating proteinuria and hypertension using ACEI and ARBs is practical and sensible. There is no consensus about the utility of more specific therapies; trials of prednisolone, plus more potent immunosuppression, fish oils and other interventions, e.g. tonsillectomy, have failed to resolve this matter.

Interstitial nephritis

Acute interstitial nephritis (AIN) is an acute, sometimes reversible, inflammatory disease diagnosed after renal biopsy. It is a relatively common cause of renal dysfunction (15% of AKI in some series). It can occur at any age, though is rarer in children. Drugs – antibiotics, nonsteroidals, allopurinol, diuretics – are frequent causes of AIN, which can also be idiopathic, secondary to Chinese herbs, other nephrotoxins, infections, collagen vascular disease and malignancy.

Presentation is with oliguria in many cases, in the context of renal impairment, which can progress rapidly. Where an allergic reaction to a drug is the reason for AIN, there can be fever, rash, arthralgia, eosinophilia-eosinophiluria, sterile pyuria. Conventional urinalysis for blood and protein can be bland.

Stopping any potentially responsible drugs and a short course of prednisolone are typical interventions. Recovery is usual, though not universal, and some residual renal impairment due to renal interstitial fibrosis secondary to the inflammation is common.

Lupus nephritis

Systemic lupus can affect the kidney. In rare cases the only manifestation of lupus is renal disease. Involvement can range from low-grade proteinuria/non-visible haematuria, through nephrotic syndrome, to fulminant AKI. Systemic lupus classically presents in premenopausal women, with hair loss, mouth ulcers, skin rash and arthralgia. More rarely, venous thrombotic episodes may herald antiphospholipid syndrome, either in isolation or as part of classic systemic lupus erythematous (SLE).

Renal lupus is diagnosed in the clinical context of SLE, with positive autoantibodies and after a renal biopsy, which is necessary to delineate the extent and severity of renal involvement. Treatment involves a combination of BP reduction, possible anticoagulation (if antiphospholipid positive) and immunosuppression (as above).

Membranous nephropathy

Membranous nephropathy (MN) is a relatively common renal lesion, and one of the leading causes of primary glomerular disease. It is found in subjects of all ages, with a peak incidence in middle to old age. It is more common in men than women. Presentation is typically with isolated proteinuria, nephrotic syndrome, hypertension and renal impairment.

MN can be idiopathic, or secondary to underlying malignancy (lung, colon, other), systemic infection, HIV, hepatitis B or C, SLE or drugs such as gold, penicillamine, nonsteroidals and others.

ACEI and ARB are used for raised BP and proteinuria. Persistent nephrotic syndrome and progressive renal impairment are indications for immunosuppression, with prednisolone and other agents such as chlorambucil, cyclophosphamide or ciclosporin.

Minimal change nephropathy

Minimal change nephropathy (MCN) is the commonest cause of nephrotic syndrome in children (70–90%) and younger adults (50%). It is diagnosed more rarely in older subjects. It is a histological diagnosis, reached after renal biopsy. In children (see Chapter 12) it is usual to treat acute-onset nephrotic syndrome with steroids, but in adults a renal biopsy is usually performed before treatment, as the differential diagnosis is wider. Primary MCN is by far the most common, but secondary MCN is known in association with viral infection, HIV, drug use and malignancy.

Presentation is typically with acute onset nephrotic syndrome (see Chapter 7). Oedema can be prodigious, and pleural and pericardial effusions and ascites can be severe.

Treatment is with oral prednisolone for many weeks (typically three months). Response rates are best in children and young adults. Relapse is not usual, though some patients relapse in a predictable fashion as steroid doses fall. Acute infections can also precipitate relapse. Other drugs, in steroid-insensitive or steroid-dependent subjects, may be needed.

Myeloma, amyloid and the kidney

Renal involvement by myeloma is quite common. This can be as a result of hypercalcaemia, hyperuricaemia, cast nephropathy, interstitial nephritis or direct infiltration by plasma cells. The presentation can be proteinuria, hypertension and renal impairment.

Immunocyte (AL) and reactive (AA) amyloid can affect the kidney, with the usual presentation being isolated proteinuria, more typically nephrotic syndrome.

Treatment of the underlying condition leading to myeloma or amyloidosis is the only specific intervention. Renal impairment can limit chemotherapy options.

Nephrotic syndrome

See Chapter 7.

Pyelonephritis

Acute pyelonephritis (AP; see Chapter 6) is infection of the renal parenchyma caused by bacterial infection ascending the urinary tract from the bladder.

Like acute cystitis, AP is much more common in women than men. Risk factors include structural abnormalities of the urinary tract, pregnancy, diabetes, asymptomatic bacteriuria, urinary tract instrumentation and sexual intercourse. In men, AP is more often seen over the age of 40, with prostatic disease and renal stones being the commonest underlying reasons.

The commonest microorganisms are *Escherichia coli*, *Proteus*, *Pseudonomas* and *Klebsiella* spp.

Patients usually present with fever, rigors, loin pain and lower urinary tract symptoms. Loin pain and tenderness can be severe. There can be septicaemic shock where there is obstruction or immunosuppression. Leucocytosis, raised C-reactive protein (CRP), urine and blood cultures can all aid diagnosis. Renal ultrasound usually shows an enlarged kidney.

Treatment is with appropriate antibiotics, administered intravenously in severe cases. Obstruction should be relieved.

Renal (ANCA-positive) vasculitis

Vasculitis can involve large blood vessels, and smaller ones. Only small vessel vasculitis commonly involves the kidney. This involvement can be anything from low-grade proteinuria/non-visible haematuria, through nephrotic syndrome, to fulminant AKI (also known as rapidly progressive glomerulonephritis, or RPGN).

This is characteristically a disease of middle-aged to older patients, though it can occur in children. Presentation can be 'renal only', i.e. no systemic vasculitis features clinically, to multiple organ/system involvement. Joint pains, myalgia, skin rash, iritis, uveitis, general malaise, anorexia and weight loss can accompany any renal manifestations.

One important association is pulmonary–renal syndromes. The lung and the kidney can be involved in vasculitis in Goodpasture's disease (acute pulmonary haemorrhage), Wegener's granulomatosis (haemoptysis, breathlessness, lung nodules on chest x-ray or CT, and often deafness and nasal blockage and epistaxis), Churg–Strauss syndrome (with asthma and eosinophilia) and lupus.

Diagnosis comes from correctly interpreting the multisystem features. Anaemia, raised white count and thrombocytosis are common. The erythrocyte sedimentation rate (ESR) and CRP are raised. More specific tests include antineutrophil cytoplasmic antibodies (ANCA).

Treatment with potent immunosuppressives (prednisolone, azathioprine, mycophenolate mofetil, cyclophosphamide, plasma exchange) can be very effective, especially if the diagnosis is made promptly, before life-threatening complications ensue. Without treatment, these diseases are often fatal.

Renovascular disease

See Chapter 8.

Thin membrane nephropathy

Persistent non-visible haematuria (see Chapter 1) is seen in around 3–5% of the UK population. Thin membrane nephropathy (TMN) is responsible for about 20–40% of this. TMN can be sporadic or, more rarely, familial. Diagnosis is made by electron microscopy of a renal biopsy specimen (measuring the width of the glomerular basement membrane, which is reduced in TMN).

This condition is usually asymptomatic, and is diagnosed on medical screening where this includes urinalysis (e.g. health/insurance medicals). Onset can be in childhood. Haematuria in TMN can be visible or non-visible, intermittent or persistent. Sometimes the visible haematuria can be painful and, very rarely, heavy enough to cause temporary ureteric or bladder obstruction. Prognosis is usually excellent.

Top Ten Tips in Kidney Disease

Satish Jayawardene[1] and David Goldsmith[2]

[1]King's College Hospital NHS Foundation Trust, London, UK
[2]King's College London, London, UK

1 Acute screen

This is usually performed if a patient has acute kidney injury (AKI) (see Chapter 2) or unexplained/newly diagnosed renal impairment. It commonly includes:

(a) ANA (antinuclear antibody).
(b) ANCA (antineutrophil cytoplasmic antibody).
(c) anti-dsDNA antibody (anti-double stranded DNA antibody).
(d) anti-GBM (glomerular basement membrane) antibody.
(e) SEP (serum electrophoresis).
(f) Serum free light chains (SFLC) OR urinary Bence-Jones proteins (BJP).
(g) Complement levels (C3 and C4).

2 Hyperkalaemia

This is commonly seen in chronic kidney disease (CKD). Measures used to treat it include:

(a) Low potassium diet: potassium is high in content in foods such as tomatoes, chocolate, nuts and orange juice. Dietetic assessment can be helpful in reducing potassium intake.
(b) Sodium bicarbonate: acidosis occurs as a consequence of decreased hydrogen ion excretion by the kidney in CKD and causes hyperkalaemia as a result of a transcellular shift. Measurement of serum bicarbonate is useful in those with CKD and supplementing it if bicarbonate concentration is < 20 mmol/L will reduce potassium concentrations. There is also some evidence that this will also slow progression of CKD (see Chapter 3).
(c) Angiotensin converting enzyme inhibitors (ACEIs)/ angiotensin II receptor blockers (ARBs)/Spironolactone/Beta-Blockers: all these drugs can increase potassium concentrations. Combining these drugs is often done in the treatment of heart failure (as well as CKD). Stopping them will contribute to lowering levels. You may need to discuss this with *both* the cardiology and the kidney teams.

(d) Loop diuretics: these will increase urinary potassium excretion (and lower plasma potassium concentration), though may exacerbate volume depletion and worsen kidney function.
(e) Calcium polystyrene sulfonate: this resin has previously been recommended for the treatment of hyperkalaemia. However, it is not appropriate for life-threatening hyperkalaemia, due to its slow onset of action. It is also associated with many gastrointestinal side-effects (especially constipation), so its use has waned in recent times.

3 Contrast nephrotoxicity (CN)

This is a form of AKI (see Chapter 2) and can occur with radio-opaque contrast used particularly for CT scans and angiograms. It is more common in those with CKD; the risk is greater the worse the stage of CKD. It usually occurs 4–7 days after exposure to contrast. Measures to prevent it include:

(a) Withholding diuretics, ACEIs and ARBs.
(b) Ensure good hydration before and after the contrast exposure. Pre-salination with sodium chloride or sodium bicarbonate is useful where patients are able to receive intravenous fluid.
(c) N-acetylcysteine: this can be used orally before and after contrast and some evidence suggests that it reduces CN.

4 Starting an ACE inhibitor +/–ARB

These drugs are used primarily as antihypertensive agents. It is essential that renal function and potassium are checked 10–14 days after their initiation. A rise in creatinine less than 30% or an estimated glomerular filtration rate (eGFR) fall of less than 25% from baseline is acceptable. Anything above this may suggest the presence of volume depletion, concurrent medications (such as nonsteroidal anti-inflammatory drugs) or renal artery stenosis.

ACEIs and ARBs are increasingly being used together to reduce proteinuria (or treat heart failure [see Tip 2] irrespective of the cause). This may lead to problems with hyperkalaemia but has been shown to provide renoprotection in those at high renal risk. If a patient develops diarrhoea and vomiting, these medications should be stopped immediately (the patients should be told to do this) and medical advice sought.

ABC of Kidney Disease, Second edition.
Edited by David Goldsmith, Satish Jayawardene and Penny Ackland.
© 2013 John Wiley & Sons, Ltd. Published 2013 by John Wiley & Sons, Ltd.

5   Change in GFR

Progressive decline in eGFR of more than 5 mL/min/1.73 m^2 within one year, or more than 10 mL/min/1.73 m^2 within five years. If this occurs, the GFR needs to be repeated. If the GFR is still reduced, or has deteriorated further, then a history and physical examination should be carried out. In particular, a careful drug history should be taken. A renal ultrasound should be performed and an acute screen sent. Emergency contact with the local renal unit should be made, particularly if the patient has AKI (see Chapter 2) with life-threatening features such as hyperkalaemia (K+ > 6.5 mmol/L), pulmonary oedema or severe acidosis (pH < 7.2).

6   Proteinuria

If a patient has proteinuria on dipstick urinalysis, this needs to be quantified with an urinary protein:creatinine ratio (PCR) or albumin:creatinine ratio (ACR). Twenty-four-hour urine collections for protein are no longer routinely performed due to the ease of collecting ACRs or PCRs (random 10–20 mL urine sample). Measurement of renal function, an acute screen and renal ultrasound should be performed if there is no apparent cause. Referral to a renal unit is recommended if proteinuria is significant (PCR > 100 mg/mmol in non-diabetics) (see Chapter 1).

7   Sudden onset of heavy proteinuria

From a background of none, or small amounts, particularly in a patient with diabetes should NOT be assumed to be diabetic in origin until proved to be so.

8   Haematuria (visible or non-visible)

All cases over the age of 40 years should be seen by an urologist for cystoscopy and urine cytology (after one episode of visible or two episodes of non-visible haematuria). A renal ultrasound, measurement of kidney function, urine PCR and an acute screen should all be performed. See Chapter 1.

9   Correcting eGFR for race

For black patients (Afro-Caribbean and African), eGFR calculated by the (Modification Diet in Renal Disease (MDRD) method should be increased by approximately 20% (multiply by 1.21).

10   Non-diabetic renal disease

About a third of diabetic patients get evidence of kidney involvement as a microvascular complication of diabetes. This is most often evidenced by progressive proteinuria, starting as micro-albuminuria, then going through proteinuria, to nephrotic-range proteinuria and loss of GFR. Typically, but not always, this is accompanied by other signs of diabetic disease, e.g. diabetic retinopathy and diabetic peripheral or autonomic neuropathy. But, especially in type 2 diabetes (much commoner than type 1), there can be associated renal problems, e.g. other drugs in use or other coexisting conditions. The absence of diabetic proliferative (laser-requiring) retinopathy does not mean the patient cannot have classic diabetic nephropathy. If the situation is not clear, or not typical in its pace of change (gradual, slow deterioration), then, if in doubt, refer to the local kidney unit or diabetic unit for advice. See 7 (sudden onest of heavy proteinuria).

Maps Showing Variation in Healthcare for People with Kidney Disease

David Goldsmith

King's College London, London, UK

The following maps are from *NHS Atlas of Variation in Healthcare for People with Kidney Disease*, 2012 (www.rightcare.nhs.uk /index.php/atlas/kidneycare). Variation could be a marker for innovative or excellent medical practice, or, perhaps more commonly, it reflects undesirable inability to match the best performing centres in terms of recognition, and timely interventions for and treatments of, chronic kidney disease.

Figure A4.1   Rate of RRT per population by country (2009; for 6 of the countries, data are not 2009).

Here, variation between nations probably reflects intrinsic prevalence of renal pathology, differential efficiencies of primary care programmes to detect and prevent renal disease, and, in some cases, potentially peverse financial incentives geared towards maximising dialysis populations.

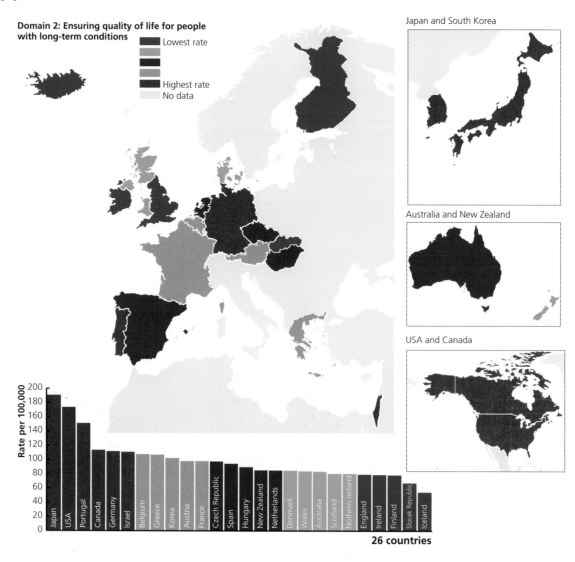

Figure A4.2 Proportion (%) of people starting RRT for CKD <90 days after presenting to renal services by renal centre (2009).

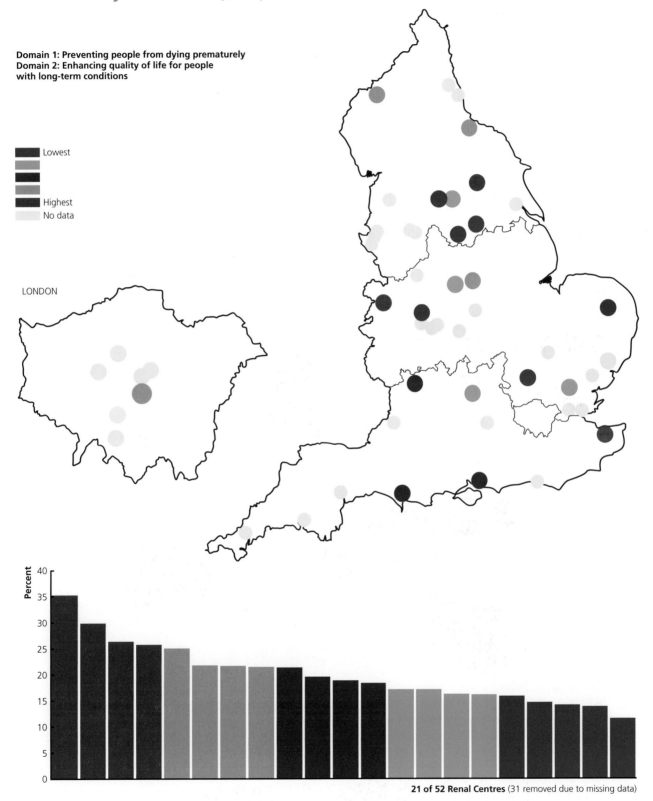

Domain 1: Preventing people from dying prematurely
Domain 2: Enhancing quality of life for people with long-term conditions

Lowest

Highest
No data

LONDON

21 of 52 Renal Centres (31 removed due to missing data)

Figure A4.3 Percentage of patients on the CKD register in whom the last blood-pressure reading, measured in the preceding 15 months, is 140/85 mmHg or less by PCT (2010/11).

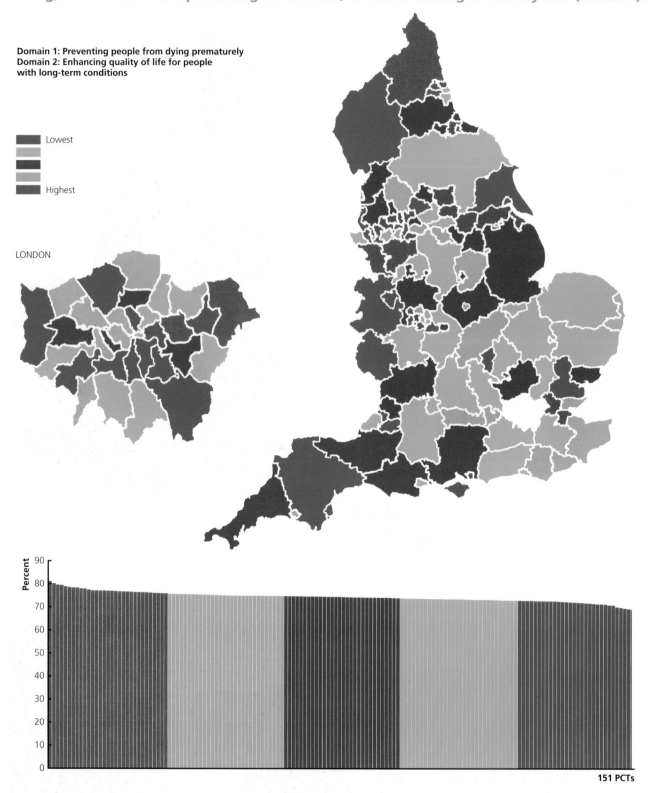

Domain 1: Preventing people from dying prematurely
Domain 2: Enhancing quality of life for people
with long-term conditions

Lowest

Highest

LONDON

151 PCTs

Figure A4.4   Percentage of patients with diabetes with a diagnosis of proteinuria or micro-albuminuria who are treated with ACEIs (or A2 antagonists) by PCT (2010/11).

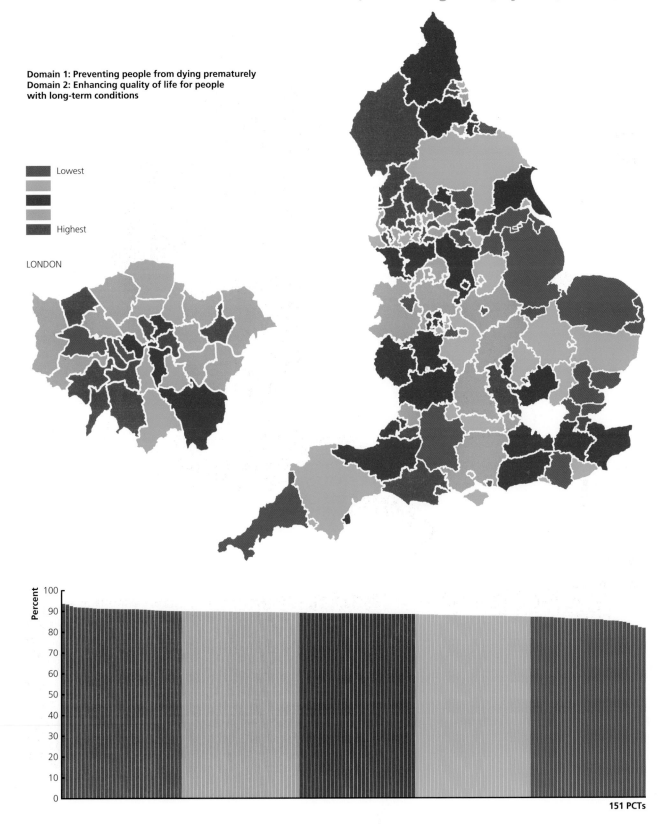

Domain 1: Preventing people from dying prematurely
Domain 2: Enhancing quality of life for people with long-term conditions

Lowest

Highest

LONDON

Index

Note: Page references in *italics* refer to Figures; those in **bold** refer to Tables and Boxes

ABC of Pain

Lesley A. Colvin & Marie Fallon
Western General Hospital, Edinburgh; University of Edinburgh

Pain is a common presentation and this brand new title focuses on the pain management issues most often encountered in primary care. *ABC of Pain*:

- Covers all the chronic pain presentations in primary care right through to tertiary and palliative care and includes guidance on pain management in special groups such as pregnancy, children, the elderly and the terminally ill
- Includes new findings on the effectiveness of interventions and the progression to acute pain and appropriate pharmacological management
- Features pain assessment, epidemiology and the evidence base in a truly comprehensive reference
- Provides a global perspective with an international list of expert contributors

JUNE 2012 | 9781405176217 | 128 PAGES | £24.99/US$44.95/€32.90/AU$47.95

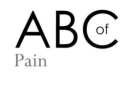
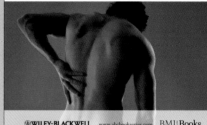

ABC of Urology

3RD EDITION

Chris Dawson & Janine Nethercliffe
Fitzwilliam Hospital, Peterborough; Edith Cavell Hospital, Peterborough

Urological conditions are common, accounting for up to one third of all surgical admissions to hospital. Outside of hospital care urological problems are a common reason for patients needing to see their GP.

- *ABC of Urology, 3rd Edition* provides a comprehensive overview of urology
- Focuses on the diagnosis and management of the most common urological conditions
- Features 4 additional chapters: improved coverage of renal and testis cancer in separate chapters and new chapters on management of haematuria, laparoscopy, trauma and new urological advances
- Ideal for GPs and trainee GPs, and is useful for junior doctors undergoing surgical training, while medical students and nurses undertaking a urological placement as part of their training programme will find this edition indispensable

MARCH 2012 | 9780470657171 | 88 PAGES | £23.99/US$37.95/€30.90/AU$47.95

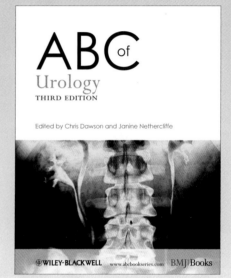

ABC series

An outstanding collection of resources for everyone in primary care

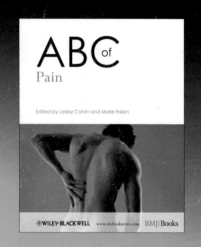

ABC of Pain

Edited by Lesley Colvin and Marie Fallon

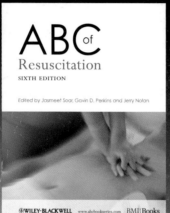

ABC of Resuscitation

SIXTH EDITION

Edited by Jasmeet Soar, Gavin D. Perkins and Jerry Nolan

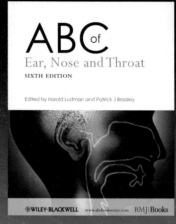

ABC of Ear, Nose and Throat

SIXTH EDITION

Edited by Harold Ludman and Patrick J Bradley

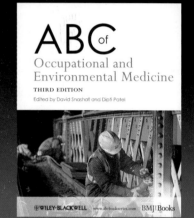

ABC of Occupational and Environmental Medicine

THIRD EDITION

Edited by David Snashall and Dipti Patel

The *ABC* series contains a wealth of indispensable resources for GPs, GP registrars, junior doctors, doctors in training and all those in primary care

▶ **Highly illustrated, informative and a practical source of knowledge**

▶ **An easy-to-use resource, covering the symptoms, investigations, treatment and management of conditions presenting in day-to-day practice and patient support**

▶ **Full colour photographs and illustrations aid diagnosis and patient understanding of a condition**

For more information on all books in the *ABC* series, including links to further information, references and links to the latest official guidelines, please visit:

www.abcbookseries.com

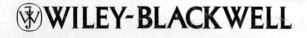

WILEY-BLACKWELL

BMJ Books